Blessings of Barrenness

How to Surrender Infertility and Pregnancy Loss

By

Christi Kari

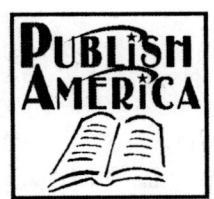

PublishAmerica
Baltimore

© 2005 by Christi Kari.

All rights reserved. No part of this book may be reproduced, stored in a retrieval system or transmitted in any form or by any means without the prior written permission of the publishers, except by a reviewer who may quote brief passages in a review to be printed in a newspaper, magazine or journal.

First printing

At the specific preference of the author, PublishAmerica allowed this work to remain exactly as the author intended, verbatim, without editorial input.

ISBN: 1-4137-7382-6
PUBLISHED BY PUBLISHAMERICA, LLLP
www.publishamerica.com
Baltimore

Printed in the United States of America

All scripture quotations, unless otherwise indicated, are taken from the THE HOLY BIBLE, NEW INTERNATIONAL VERSION®. NIV®. Copyright © 1973, 1978, 1984 by International Bible Society. Used by permission of Zondervan. All rights reserved.

Holy Bible, New Living Translation, copyright © 1996 by Tyndale Charitable Trust. All rights reserved. Scripture quotations marked (NLT) are taken from the Holy Bible, New Living Translation, copyright © 1996. Used by permission of Tyndale House Publishers, Inc., Wheaton, Illinois 60189. All rights reserved.

This book is dedicated to my mother, Lynn Hockersmith, who introduced me to Jesus while I was a small child. Mom, you have always been my biggest "cheerleader" and your unconditional love and encouragement has given me the courage to believe I can do whatever I put my mind to. Thank you!

Thank you also to Cindi McMenamin, Nicole Henderson and Shane Thomas for helping make this book come to fruition.

Table of Contents

Introductory Poem

1. What You Need to Know First	13
2. My Story—Establishing Faith Through Trials	23
Experiencing the "i" Word	
Cultivating Faith	
3. Hannah's Story—Developing a Relationship with Christ	45
Feeling Empty	
Getting to Know Christ	
4. Rebekah's Story—Reading the Bible and Praying Daily	65
Developing a Habit of Reading God's Word Daily	
Learning How to Pray	
5. Sarah's Story—Identifying Unconfessed Sin	83
Meeting the "Lion"	
Exposing the Idols of Obsession, Pride and Pity	
6. Elizabeth's Story—Surrendering Your Plans	111
Surrendering Your Will for God's Will	
Waiting on God's Perfect Timing	
7. Manoah's Wife's Story—Acknowledging People or Things on God's Throne	131
Making God Your First Priority	
Allowing Your Husband to be Head of the Household	
8. Rachel's Story—Humbling Yourself Unto the Lord	149
Being Humble When You Feel Broken	
Being Prepared for Insensitive Remarks and Suggestions	
Attending Child-Centered Occasions	
9. Stacie's Story—Opening Your Mind to Other Plans God Has for You	177
Dealing with Pregnancy Loss	
Enlightening Family and Friends About Infertility	
Talking Before You Test	
Considering Adoption	
10. Karen's Story—Opening Your Eyes to Abundant Blessings	223
Grieving is a Process	
Blessing You is God's Gift	
Moving on as a Complete Family	
11. Christine's Story—Feeling Desperate for God	255
Keeping up Your Shield	
Examining Your Purpose for Living	
Blessings in Disguise	
Notes	271
Appendix A: Resources	277
Appendix B: Spiritual Gifts Questionnaire	290
Appendix C: Answers to fill-in-the blank verses	299

Introductory Poem

When I reflect upon the 10-year heartache I experienced with infertility, I would describe it as a wild, sporadic, out-of-control chase. This poem personifies the highs and lows barren women go through, as well as the end result God has in store for each of us—joy! No one will relate to it but us.

Infertility: "The Chase"

Walking alone in the desert. Dry, barren, dusty, trail beneath my feet.
See object—a bunny so sweet, so cuddly. Want it! Walk toward him.
He scampers away. See it—start to chase him. Rabbit rounds a big rock.
Peek around rock, it's gone! Round the rock running aimlessly.
Where is it? Running, chasing—no bunny in sight. Tired. Weak.
Frustrated. Pick up the pace. Trip. Fall. Get up… brush off dust. Start out slowly.
See rabbit. It's right there. Increase speed. Trip again. Skin knee.
Sadness. Pain. Get back on trail. Looking, seeking, desperate.
See tip of bunny tail. Finally! Run faster. It hides. It alludes. Breathing hard.
Panic! Racing. Can't keep up. Round the bend. See it. There he is.
So pure, so supple. Reach, grab— got it!! Look down, rabbit is gone.
Only an illusion—a puff of smoke! Disbelief. Disappointment. Feeling foolish.
Snake suddenly slithers up. Slimy. Shifty. Sneaky. Belly in the shape of a bunny.
"You want it?" he rasps. *"Take it, it's yours. Be mine, be happy."*
Something's not right. Evil looms. But bunny in plain sight! Want it.
Reach out.
Bush suddenly shakes. *"Don't be fooled, it's a trick,"* it warns.
Snake and rabbit disappear. A vapor. Bush says, *"Do not be afraid, you are not alone."* Lie down under bush. Sheltered from the sun.
Feeling protected.
Fall asleep. Start to dream. Hear a cry—a baby! He's alone and helpless.
Pick up infant. Smell its tender scent. Heart pounding. Raise baby to sky.
Shout *"thank you!"* to the heavens. *"God is good! God is love!"*
Baby vanishes. Arms still in the air. Cry out *"God is peace!"*

You see, God's "will" may or may not include a baby for you, however, what He has planned for you is bigger than anything you could have dreamed of or imagined.[1] As you go through this trial, allow Him to grace you with His love and His peace as He patiently teaches you what your true identity is. To the Creator of the universe, you are not broken, you are perfect just the way you are.[2]

Christi

A Special Note to Friends and Loved Ones

If you have an infertile woman in your life either through medical challenges, pregnancy loss, secondary infertility (having one or more child and being unable to conceive again), or through the evidence of her husband's sterility, you might notice her acting "differently." Perhaps she's moody, maybe she's avoiding you or others, or she may be acting a little crazy. The point is this trial is bigger than life to her.

She wants answers and she wants them NOW. Because the answers generally come over a lengthy span of time, the waiting and wondering nearly drive her insane. You can encourage her by learning about her battle and by implementing the advice offered in this book. See Chapter 9 for suggestions and advice.

Chapter 1–What You Need to Know First

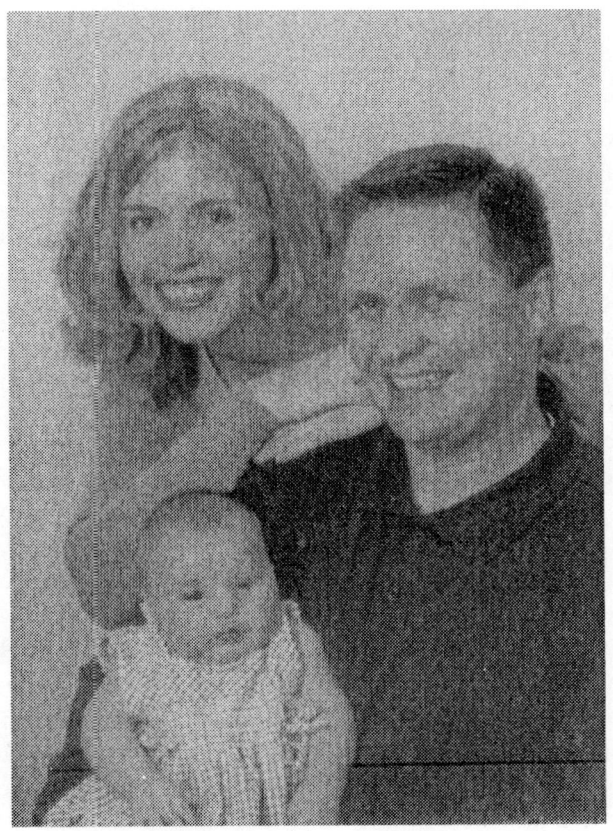

Sheri, Matthew and Brooke

-Learning About Your Self
-Taking a Deep Look at Your Faith
-Trying to Understand Your World
-Surrendering Your Suffering

Chapter 1–What You Need to Know First

I applaud you for picking up this book and opening it. It is very difficult to broach the idea of one's fertility, let alone entertain the thought there may be a problem. For me, the "problem" became a nightmare; it was new and foreign and eventually it became the "i" word —my opponent.

If it is new to you too, let's make sure we are "on the same page" by looking at the definitions of infertility. *Primary infertility* is the inability to conceive after at least one year of unprotected intercourse, or the inability to successfully carry a child to live birth. *Secondary infertility* is the inability to conceive or successfully give birth to a child multiple times.

My "inability to conceive" was never rectified, hence my 10-year struggle included anger, obsession, denial, pride and loneliness. I searched for people and resources to aid me in my out-of-control journey to no avail. After enduring years of testing, I finally learned how to surrender *my* plan, and almost immediately a 3-week-old baby girl was placed in my arms by a selfless birth mother. Two years later, another loving woman chose to place her day-old baby boy in my awaiting arms.

Although my heart was so full, I still felt heartache for my friends and acquaintances whose arms were empty. With the help of the Holy Spirit, I wrote a Bible study and subsequent "care group" for these ladies. Several of them told me later that it was very, very difficult to call and sign up. One lady spent 30 minutes in the driveway trying to conjure up the courage to enter my home for the study. I understood and I'm willing to bet you can relate as well. Admitting there may be a problem is the first step to working through this trial.

Because I have a heart for ladies and families going through infertility, I felt led to expand the Bible study into this book. It draws upon my own experiences, as well as the journeys of the 20 women who participated in the care group. You will be reading testimonies from them and you will also benefit from the many, many conversations I've had with women over the years and their stories of God's healing.

There are four ways this book is intended to help you. You will learn about: 1) your self, 2) your faith, 3) your world, and 4) your suffering. By taking a serious look at these four areas of your life, you will gain a better understanding of your beliefs and expectations and you will gain a wealth of practical advice and spiritual guidance. Next, you must choose to absorb this material and put into daily practice.

Remind yourself that many of us have walked in your shoes and come out on the other side—some with the prize originally anticipated; others with a broader understanding of a different reward intended for them. Yet all of us emerged with peace of mind, renewed joy, and hope for eternity spent with the Author of Life.

Learning About Your Self

If you're like me, when you reached the point in your life when you were ready to conceive, you just expected it to happen. Because something so natural didn't happen, it's normal to experience feelings of disappointment, inadequacy, embarrassment, devastation, bitterness and even shame.

There may be times when you feel like you are losing your mind. I want to reassure you that you're probably reacting to this huge issue just like the rest of us did. I will be the first to admit that experiencing infertility is devastating. It's a very serious and sensitive issue. This is how one woman described her struggle:

I know that understanding infertility is difficult; there are times when it seems even I don't understand. This struggle has provoked intense and unfamiliar feelings in me and I fear that my reactions to these feelings may be misunderstood. You may describe me this way: obsessed, moody, helpless, depressed, envious, too serious, obnoxious, aggressive, antagonistic, and cynical. These aren't very admirable traits; no wonder your understanding of my infertility is difficult. I prefer to describe me this way: confused, rushed and impatient, afraid, isolated and alone, guilty and ashamed, angry, sad and hopeless, and unsettled.

You are taking the first step of healing by reading this book. Take your time as you read it and consider each point even if it doesn't seem to relate to you at first. There is a great likelihood that some things will sound harsh to you or offensive. I apologize in advance. Just keep reading and I'm sure you will eventually grasp the concept I am trying to convey.

Notice there are question and answer pages that introduce each chapter

CHAPTER 1—WHAT YOU NEED TO KNOW FIRST

and Bible verses that correspond to them. Take the time to sit down and answer the questions *before* you read each chapter. Be truthful. Search your heart for the answers. Ask God to "fill you with His Holy Spirit" so that you can converse back and forth with Him. Give Him quiet time to talk to you and soothe you. Notice that in some cases, I have given you examples to stimulate your thoughts.

Use this book. Allow it to be as interactive as possible. Underline points that you want to refer back to. Highlight encouraging verses. Personalize this book and allow it to aid you during this tumultuous journey.

Also, take any Bible verses that encourage you and place them somewhere you will read often. You can write them in lipstick on your bathroom mirror. You can tape them to the dashboard of your car (just be careful not to cover up the gas gauge or speedometer). If you prefer something fancier, decorate them on your computer and place the printouts on your refrigerator. I am confident these verses will inspire and cheer you on each time you look at them.

Taking a Deep Look at Your Faith

I mentioned earlier that I sought out help because I felt so alone. Quite often, loneliness becomes a barren woman's best friend. In my humanity, I started to focus on what I didn't have – that illusive baby – and God's blessings that surrounded me were overlooked. My eyes had been completely removed from the Lord, and I fell into a trap – obsession with motherhood.

When this foothold gave way to a stronghold, I put my trust in myself and the medical community, instead of the Lord. Additionally, I began to question my faith in God who promised to give me my "heart's desires." Does this sound familiar to you? From what I've witnessed, many infertile women fall into these same traps. For most barren women, myself included, the stronghold turns into bondage and we:

- Fall into an extremely unhealthy and down-spiraling "pity party."
- Start praying for "our will" instead of God's perfect will.
- Grow incredibly impatient and refuse to wait for God's perfect timing.
- Put our focus on pregnancy and forget about our marriage and the needs of our husband.
- Abandon friends and family members who have children and force our selves into seclusion.

- Lash out at friends, family members and strangers with children.
- Refuse to attend anything related to babies or children such as church, baby showers, parks, family gatherings, etc.

The very best advice I can offer you is to develop a strong and precious relationship with Jesus Christ. I understand that you may be feeling let down or even angry with God right now, however, believe it or not, this trial is intended to strengthen your relationship with Him. He alone will bless you with the peace and strength to get through this period and understand that His plan for you is in your best interests.

If you are a "hard core" Christian, a new believer, or if you are seeking the One, true God, I am confident this book will help you cope with the heartache, grief, loneliness and desperation of infertility. We will look at your true motives for motherhood and we will discuss the grieving process.

You will walk away with a better perspective of God's plan for your life and you will be better prepared to handle thoughtless advice from well-meaning friends and family, as well as uncomfortable situations such as baby showers, Mother's Day and other child-centered holidays and occasions.

You will learn about your true identity when you read some of the "love letters" God wrote to you. You will learn how reading the Bible and praying daily will make this struggle an intimate adventure with your heavenly Father. Ultimately, you will recognize that by surrendering your will and your timing for God's, He will bless you beyond your wildest dreams.

Trying to Understand Your World

Unless you are fortunate enough to have a support group in your life, you probably feel left out right now. Being infertile taught me what it feels like to be in the minority. I want to give you an example of what I'm saying by drawing an illustration. Let me ask you something: What do the majority of women love to do when they get together, besides eating? The answer is: They love to swap birthing stories. I am certain it's been going on since the day another woman entered the earth and sat down for a chat with Eve. Somehow "the chat" becomes some sort of twisted contest to determine who was the bravest, who endured the pain without the use of drugs, who had the longest labor, and who gave birth to the largest baby. Here is a fairly typical scenario—see if it sounds familiar to you:

CHAPTER 1—WHAT YOU NEED TO KNOW FIRST

*Today I sit with my friends and wince as one after another, they exchange gory stories of ripping, episiotomies and afterbirth. Visions swirl inside my head as I try to picture each woman in the room writhing in pain, swearing and clutching their husbands' hands as descriptions of childbirth are described in great detail. I envision them looking their worst as sweat drips from their foreheads and their legs are outstretched...when suddenly, my thoughts are interrupted as a blond across the room asks me to share **my** "childbirth story."*

I'm caught off guard. I'm unexpectedly in the spotlight. My eyes scan the room for the nearest exit as I plan my escape. My face feels 350 degrees; is it as red as it feels? My hands are sweaty as I wring them together. What do I say? Ideas race trough my mind as I search for a witty reply.

Finally, my mouth wrenches open like an oyster being robbed of its precious pearl. The words, 'I don't have one' barely squeak out of my mouth as though I am whispering a shameful secret. 'What do you mean?' asks the redhead seated next to me. 'Haven't you been married six years? What's the problem?' she probes. 'Don't you want to have children?'

All eyes are on me as the group waits for a reply. I feel like 'loser' has just been stamped on my forehead. Now I really want to run away. Why does she have to be so hurtful to me I wonder. I want to pretend that I don't know these ladies and I'll never see them again. As they sense my discomfort, some of them start to fidget in their chairs. The uneasy looks on their faces change from curiosity to pity. I hate that look!

The next thing I know, they'll be telling me to stand on my head after intercourse, or the sure fire way to conceive – go on a cruise. Or even worse, to stop trying so hard and adopt. Then I'm sure to become pregnant! Why is this happening to me? Why not Fran, the lady who lives down my street with six kids and different fathers for each? She doesn't even appreciate those precious babies. I could do a much better job as their mother I'm sure!

This scenario is real to me and possibly to you. I have sat through many of these sessions before. I got so tired of hearing my friends rambling about their kids. If they weren't talking about childbirth, the conversations centered around characters in kids shows that I didn't recognize; soccer game schedules; or ballet recitals. It was so frustrating. I couldn't find it in my heart to be happy for them. All I could think about was their inconsideration and my isolation.

If you have undergone pregnancy loss, this kind of chat session is especially hurtful. Those of you who are experiencing secondary infertility may share your story with a smile, although the ladies in the room are unaware of your secret sadness.

The truth of the matter is, during my long struggle with infertility, I took my eyes off the Lord and placed them on myself. I was too busy focusing on "me, me, me." Here's the proof. Look back at the illustration I just shared. Start counting at the beginning of the italicized illustration and see how many times the words "I," "I'm," "my," and "me" are used. The answer is an astounding 43 times!

When we refocus our eyes on our Creator, where they belong, perhaps sad stories like this can be avoided. That's easier said than done, I know! Instead of surrendering this struggle to the Lord, I chose to wallow in self-pity and disappointment for 10 long years. I fully understand any feelings of disappointment, anger and frustration you may be feeling. My heart aches for you and I implore you to implement the advice I will be sharing so that you can avoid the mistakes I made.

Surrendering Your Suffering

While suffering through this trial, I skipped right over what God wanted for me and spent much of the journey just wanting to know "why?" I was obsessed with questions such as: *Why is God allowing me to go through such misery? Why me? Why won't my reproductive parts work right? Why does it have to hurt so bad?* No one had answers for me, not even my doctors. I wish I had known about James 1:2-4 back then:

> *"Consider it pure joy, my brothers, whenever you face trials of many kinds, because you know that the testing of your faith develops perseverance. Perseverance must finish its work so that you may be mature and complete, not lacking anything."*

Here is the answer: Only God knows why. He sends trials because he is a loving Father who longs to nurture our faith and create a closer relationship between us and Him. Perhaps if I had been aware of this I would have made the best of it instead of kicking and screaming through it all. Because so many women react the way I did and ask the same questions, I have spent a lot of time thinking about this and have come up with 10 ways God uses infertility to accomplish His purposes. This is what I have found:

CHAPTER 1—WHAT YOU NEED TO KNOW FIRST

1. A barren womb is disguised as a "trial" designed to test your faith and train you in perseverance and confidence which will ultimately result in pure joy.
2. A barren womb is designed to strengthen your relationship with your Father above and introduce you to the saving power of His Son, Jesus Christ.
3. A barren womb forces you to trust in the Lord, dig deep into His Word, and learn to pray for strength, obedience and wisdom daily.
4. A barren womb helps you identify unconfessed sin in your life that results in unanswered prayer and separation from the guidance and protection of your heavenly Father.
5. A barren womb teaches you to surrender your will and your timing for God's perfect will and His timing.
6. A barren womb makes you aware of people, objects or addictions that "sit on the throne" of your life–a place reserved for God only.
7. A barren womb forces you to humble yourself unto the Lord by eliminating unforgiveness, jealousy and anger.
8. A barren womb opens your mind to other plans God has for you… plans to prosper you in ways other than your own.
9. A barren womb opens your eyes to blessings all around you, especially your husband and your marriage.
10. A barren womb forces you to examine your purpose for living.

Through the stories of barren women from the Bible and contemporary women as well, we will look at how these ladies handled their trials and how God's purposes were accomplished. I want to note that in describing what I call the "Bible's Barren Society," I took the liberty of describing the events in contemporary, narrative form and I truly hope it is not offensive to you.

Pay careful attention and learn from others' experiences. I am confident that out of all the "stories" in this book, at least one will captivate you and possibly even convict you. If you are the competitive type, experiences listed in this book will equip you to treat this trial as a challenge so you will come out of it victorious. If you are more passive in your personality, this information will give you the courage and perseverance you will need to fight this battle.

You would be wise to always keep in mind how deeply God loves you. He's not picking on you—again, the end result that He wants for you is joy. He alone can enlighten you on why he chose this particular trial for you and what he is trying to reveal to and through you. It is possible that you will have to wait awhile, however, I guarantee that if you allow God to teach you perseverance, and the patience to wait and surrender your plans for His, your joy will surely come!

Because

Why? Why? Why?
we simply don't understand.
How? How? How?
could this be happening to me?
What? What? What?
have I done?
Who? Who? Who?
is responsible for this crisis?
When? When? When?
will it all be over?
Please! Please! Please!
somebody help me.

Dianne Fossett 3/03/03
Used with permission

"So now, since we have been made right in God's sight by faith in his promises, we can have real peace with him because of what Jesus Christ our Lord has done for us. For because of our faith, he has brought us into this place of highest privilege where we now stand, and we confidently and joyfully look forward to actually becoming all that God has in mind for us to be." **Romans 5:1-2 (NLT)**

Chapter Two—Establishing Faith Through Trials

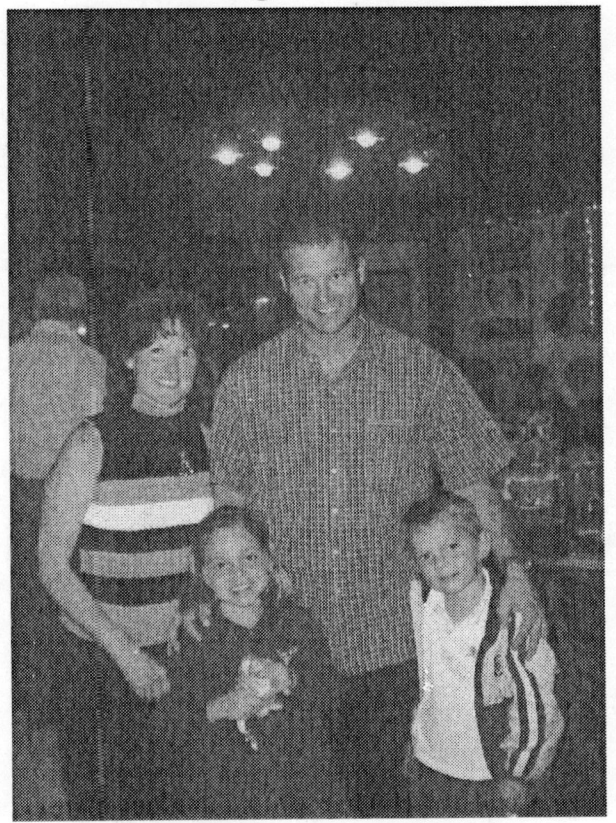

Christi, Shawn, Alexis and Jesse

-Experiencing The "i" Word
    Admitting Denial
    Filling the "Void"
    Realizing Your Sincere Motives
-Cultivating Faith
    Trials "Grow You Up" in Faith
    Fear Steals Your Joy
    Peace is a "Heart Thing"

Chapter Two–Establishing Faith Through Trials

1. Describe the point in your life when you felt ready to start a family. How did you feel? (Excited? Nervous? Apprehensive? Ready?)

_____

_____

_____

2. What were your reasons for wanting to expand your family and why did you choose that period of time?

_____

_____

_____

3. If you have a child or children and you are unable to conceive again, describe your emotions and desires to procreate again:

_____

_____

_____

4. In the beginning, what were your husband's reasons for wanting to become a father?

_____

_____

_____

5. Was he prepared to become a father? Yes or No? (Circle one.) If not, did you forge ahead without regard to his desires? Yes or No? If you are experiencing secondary infertility, is your husband as disappointed as you are? Yes or No? Have you asked him about his feelings? Yes or No?

6. If you have been dealing with infertility for a long period of time, have your reasons for wanting a child changed? Yes or No? If so, what are they now?

_____

_____

_____

7. Are you shocked or did you subconsciously suspect a problem could arise? Has anyone in your family experienced infertility? Please elaborate on both questions:

_____

_____

_____

8. Could you be infertile and experiencing denial? Yes or No? If so, how long do you intend to remain there?

_____

_____

_____

9. How do you fill the "void" in your life? (Drugs? Alcohol? Promiscuousness? Overeating? Over exercising? Excessive shopping? Reading the Bible? Praying?)

_____

_____

_____

10. What are your *real* fears regarding infertility?

_____

_____

_____

Recommended Reading:

Daniel 12:10
Jeremiah 29:11-13
John 14:27, 16:33
2 Corinthians 4:17, 5:7
2 Timothy 1:7
1 Peter 1:6-7, 4:12

Psalm 37:4, 71:1, 73:28
Matthew 22:37, 39
Romans 5:1-5
Philippians 4:6-7, 13
James 1:2-7, 12
1 John 4:18

Look up these verses and fill in the blanks:

2 Chronicles 16:9a: *"For the eyes of the Lord range throughout the earth to _____ those whose hearts are _____ committed to him."*

2 Corinthians 12:10: *"Since I know it is all for Christ's good, I am quite content with my weaknesses and with insults, hardships, persecutions, and calamities. For when I am _____, then I am _____."*

"Why *do I have to go through this?"*
Answer #1—A barren womb is disguised as a "trial" designed to test your faith and train you in perseverance and confidence which will ultimately result in pure joy.

Chapter 2–My Story

Growing up on the plains of Kansas, I enjoyed playing trucks in the dusty dirt, as well as football and baseball with my two brothers and the area country boys. As time went by, I caught up with two local schoolgirls and my creative time was spent inside with dollies, a tea set, and my Easy Bake Oven®.

I remember clearly riding home on the big, yellow school bus gleefully singing, 'First comes love, then comes marriage, then comes the baby in the baby carriage,' over and over with my little girlfriends. We submerged ourselves in fairy tales; one in particular was about a princess held up in a castle awaiting her prince to save her so they could live happily ever after.

I was that princess. We had a tight-knit family and my parents made me feel loved unconditionally. My face usually beamed with a smile and I believed everything people told me—'gullible' and 'naïve' are adjectives many people used to describe me.

My best friend and I actually took time in high school to write down plans for our dream weddings complete with drawings of our lacey gowns. Throughout the years, teachers admonished my daydreaming – thoughts of being a 'mommy' someday filled my visions. During high school, my list of favorite names for babies changed sporadically as newer and more creative ones came along. Megan, Mason, Amanda and Joseph topped the list when I flew the nest and went off to college.

It was there, at the university, that I met my prince. His name was Shawn and he was the most upright, goal-oriented, Christian man I had ever met. The attraction was instantaneous and the desire to give up my lifestyle of partying, *drinking, and dating happened practically overnight.*

We married one year later and after we both graduated, he started veterinary school, a four-year degree. Because I had to work and would have no means for childcare, procreation had to be put off. Finally, during his last year of school, I happily threw the contraceptives away and just expected to become pregnant within a year. It was a natural expectation considering I come from a very large, fertile family.

Four years later, I wasn't pregnant. I was now 30 years old, married for nine years and childless. It just didn't make sense. My feelings ranged from devastation, to inadequacy and shame. My feelings of shame were so overwhelming that I couldn't say the word 'infertility' or even think I could possibly fall into such a 'category.' The 'i' word became my adversary for 120 months!

Finally, in 1992 I started documenting my temperature daily and using ovulation kits to aid doctors in testing procedures. It was a very lonely time. My husband did what was required, but his heart was not in it. He had finally accomplished his goal and was practicing veterinary medicine. His work filled 16 hours of his day and he didn't appreciate coming home to a whining wife.

Once I had my laparoscopy (you will read about this surgery in Chapter 9), the doctors gave me three months to become pregnant. It didn't happen and I was crushed. I just didn't have it in me to endure fertility drugs or the expense and emotional roller coaster of further testing such as In Vitro Fertilization or Artificial Insemination.

I wanted a guarantee. So, I decided adoption would be best for us. Looking back, it was absurd that I made such a big decision on my own and tried to force this alternative on my husband. My tunnel vision should have been directed to my marriage instead of motherhood. Of course, my husband said 'no' as I pleaded and begged him to adopt, so my anger was replaced with bitterness and resentment.

Obsession filled my days and nights and then pride reared its ugly head. I wasn't about to expose my inadequacy to others, so I put on a facade of cheerfulness. Eventually, God had a close friend wipe that mask right off my face and the protective walls I had so carefully built crumbled around me.

It was very confusing, however, God had finally broken me down and was able to direct me down the course He had planned for me. Two years later, out of the blue, my husband told me he was ready to adopt! I couldn't get us to the adoption agency fast enough!

The process took another year and I finally connected with God again. We were selected by a birth mother and the big day finally came. Our baby girl had been born and our agency directed us to drive to the hospital to pick her up. Off we went, our brand new station wagon complete with infant car seat and diaper bag, when my husband's beeper went off. It was our social worker—the birth mother had changed her mind.

Once again I was devastated. Shawn went back to work and I drove home by myself. Sitting on the edge of our bed for hours, I wrestled back and forth with the idea of suicide. In my depression I was easy prey for the enemy as he filled me with thoughts like: *You can't do anything right – no one is going to give a loser like you a baby! You should just end your misery so your husband can marry someone else and have kids of his own.*

I listened to those lies for too long and then my king came to the rescue. The Holy Spirit whispered Ephesians 1:11 (NLT) in my ear, '*...because of what Christ has done we have become gifts to God that he delights in, for as part of God's sovereign plan we were chosen from the beginning to be his, and all things happen just as he decided long ago.*' I believed that verse and I got up off that bed and moved on with my life.

It wasn't long after when I was asked to give my 'infertility testimony' at a Bible study for our church. I declined saying that I wasn't going to give a depressing talk with an even more depressing ending. However, the Holy Spirit spoke to me again and prompted me, even to the point of conviction, to give that testimony.

It was one of the hardest things I've ever done. I exposed myself to the bitter core that day. My pride was peeled away like a banana. My words must have been difficult for the audience of women to decipher through the tears and wailing. How humiliating... how humbling... how exhausting. God finally stripped me of myself and because of my surrender that day on that stage I had the baby girl God intended for me to mother in my arms one week later.

For 10 years I had asked God for a miracle and He gave it to me, but it was according to His will and His timing, not mine. He had to combat the idols in my life, such as pride, bitterness, resentment and anger. God wanted to be my ultimate desire; He wanted to be the One for whom I was desperate.

Two years later a birth mother changed her mind again before we left the driveway to pick up our son. By now my faith was much stronger and it was a little easier to take. Because of our continued trust in the Lord, five months later He blessed us with the son he had predestined us to parent. Even though it didn't seem like it at times, God certainly knew what He was doing all along!

> **"That is why, for Christ's sake, I delight in weaknesses, in insults, in hardships, in persecutions, in difficulties. For when I am weak, then I am strong." 2 Corinthians 12:10**

CHAPTER 2—ESTABLISHING FAITH THROUGH TRIALS

Experiencing The "i" Word

Unless infertility runs in your family, you were probably as shocked as I was after a year or so of unprotected intercourse and no pregnancy. Many of the ladies I have spoken with over the years have given birth to one and even two children and then experienced secondary infertility. It's just as strange and unexpected to them. My heart goes out to my friends who planned children with their husbands only to find out later that he was sterile, and to those who have experienced miscarriage or loss.

I will start out talking about infertility in general. In my testimony, I said the following: *"I was now 30 years old, married for nine years and childless. It just didn't make sense. My feelings ranged from devastation, to inadequacy and shame. My feelings of shame were so overwhelming that I couldn't say the word 'infertility' or even think I could possibly fall into such a 'category'. The 'i' word became my adversary."*

I was afraid to say the "i" word because I didn't want to label myself. I couldn't stand admitting failure. Now I sit and wonder "failure of what?" I was no less of a woman. I was no less of a wife. I was the same daughter, sister and friend I had always been. There is no reason for you to feel ashamed either. Shame is feeling guilty about something; or feeling embarrassed or disgraced. I felt guilty because I couldn't give my husband a child. Looking back, I realize that was absurd. I had no control over the predicament I was in.

The problem is God's enemy wants you and me to feel disgraced so we will give up on any inclination of being the person the Lord created us to be. Be wise and remind yourself of God's love poured out in his Word (the Bible). God created us and He desires to have a relationship with His children. Stop. Look at those first three words again: *"God created us..."*

In the Book of Genesis, Our Heavenly Father designed man in His own image because He desired to have a relationship with human beings. He gave Adam a wife and they were told to multiply the earth. Once I understood this, I realized how natural it is for us to desire to create children of our own.

Now stop and think about the last 10 words in the sentence we considered above: *"...and He desires to have a relationship with His children."* Each and everyone of us is barren for a reason; I am convinced of that. Only God knows what it is and I believe He will reveal it to you – hopefully through the one of the 10 reasons listed in this book. We are looking at the first reason – *establishing faith through trials*. To have faith in God, you must first have a *relationship* with Him.

In 1 Corinthians 11:3, we are told to keep our priorities on this earth straight. They are listed in this order: God *first* in your life, spouse *second* in priority, children (or the desire for them) *third*, career *fourth*, and self last. When God is "first" in your life that means he is at the wheel. He is steering the course of your life and you submit to Him. By humbling yourself to His control, you will reap His blessings, His protection and His peace. When you take over the wheel and try to steer your own course, you will lose out on blessings or crash because you can't see the big picture like He can.

For example, if you center all of your attention on getting pregnant and providing your husband with a child, you may neglect your marriage and lose it all. Or, if you take your eyes off of the Lord and focus on yourself and what you don't have, you miss out on His blessings and an intimate friendship with Him, therefore, you miss out on the peace that will help you get through this difficult time.

Admitting Denial

Now that we've established how completely natural it is to desire children, let's talk about denial. For me, fear initiated a vicious cycle whereby I would deny there was a problem and feeling lonely and confused I would wait for a miracle. When the blessing didn't come, my mind would revisit the idea that something could be wrong and so on. Sounds like denial to me!

In the introductory poem, "*The Chase*," I mentioned how the bunny eludes us as we chase it down the trail. Now the figurative rabbit has us hot on his trail as we wind and weave through the symbolic desert searching and chasing. No bunny in sight, we become tired, weak and frustrated. We pick up the pace only to trip and fall.

This part of the poem exemplifies the highs and lows of the illusive pregnancy. The "high" of convincing yourself you are pregnant and the "low" you experience in the toilet a day or two later. Have you found that you can convince yourself this is *the* month? I was the queen of that illusion. Every single month for 10 years I felt nauseous and bloated and if my period was a day or two late, I knew my miracle had finally come.

Off to the store I would race to purchase a home pregnancy test. In retrospect, I was setting myself up for a huge let down. When my period did come, I would spiral down into depression. My mind was filled with questions such as: *How can this be happening to me? I am a good person. I know I will be a great mother. It's not like I'm an unmarried teenager looking for a 'baby doll.' Is this some kind of sick joke?*

There were no answers and there was no one to turn to. My pastor tried, but couldn't reassure me. My mother wanted desperately to take my pain away. My

CHAPTER 2—ESTABLISHING FAITH THROUGH TRIALS

husband was too wrapped up in his career to "hold my hand," all of my friends had children, so I settled for denial. If I denied this problem, maybe the ache would go away. I could just ignore what was happening and pretend like everything was alright.

A friend of mine named Gail experienced infertility for 10 years as well; she settled for denial too. During a conversation we had, she mentioned that she decided not to have children at a fairly young age because her sisters were pregnant at the ages of 16 and 17. She changed her mind at the age of 21 when she married an older man who wanted kids. A year went by and Gail wasn't pregnant, so she visited a doctor who performed a hysterosalpingogram and a laparoscopy *(you will read about this test and surgery in Chapter 9).*

A second doctor performed other tests, as well as an endometrial biopsy only to refer her to a specialist. Gail admits, *"I was not ready to consider adoption because I was still in denial that I couldn't get pregnant.*

During this time, my sisters and even my stepmother were having children left and right. I remember just losing it once at my sister's house. My husband was holding my sister's little baby girl in a recliner. I felt like such a failure. I ran into the bedroom and just burst into tears. I asked God many times: Why me? What did I do that made me unable to have children? I begged Him to help me understand! It was a very difficult time in my life," she confided.

Denial is refusing to accept or believe. Look at the following list and if anything applies to you, talk to your husband about seeking fertility testing. Perhaps it is time to take action. (If it is, be sure to read suggestions in Chapter 9 titled "Talking Before You Test.") It is time to move from denial to action if:

- You have been unable to conceive after at least one year of unprotected intercourse or you have been unable to successfully carry a child to live birth.
- You have been unable to conceive or give birth to a child after having carried at least one pregnancy to term.
- You have irregular periods, extremely painful periods or no periods at all.
- You have a history of problems with your reproductive organs such as cysts, tubal pregnancies, etc.
- You suspect your husband could possibly be sterile (due to a childhood injury or illness).
- You are in your late 30's or early 40's and suspect a problem with fertility could arise.
- Infertility runs in your family or your husband's.

Now, look back at the questions at the beginning of this chapter. Look specifically at how you answered questions eight and nine. Are you, or have you been in denial? How long are you going to allow yourself to deny this integral part of your life? How did (or do), you handle the "void" in your life? You would be wise to ask your husband and close friends how they perceive your disposition. Ask them specific questions such as: *Do I seem agitated to you? Am I speaking positively or do I seem negative or depressed? Do I seem to focus on this void in my life too much?*

Sometimes we don't even realize how our demeanor effects others until we ask. I caution you – only ask these questions if you are prepared for the truth and also avoid asking others for suggestions on how you should handle this difficult time unless they are experiencing infertility too.

I've witnessed couples putting off testing for years and years, in fact, I did it myself. I thought that if I went to a doctor for assistance, that meant I was admitting the "i" word which to me was analogous to defeat. In retrospect, my denial wasted valuable time and wasn't healthy. How can you help yourself if you refuse to recognize a problem? How can you use this trial to better your life and give glory to God if you reject it? Find out what's really going on in your heart, in your life, and in your body (or your husband's), and keep learning more about yourself day by day.

Emotions

That time of month
is when the ache
fills your heart the most.
Hormones whirling
Emotions twirling,
All kinds of thoughts are spinning in your head.
Our feelings are so intense,
Our emotions are so high.
The ache for the child
we do not hold
becomes almost unbearable.
Each month, that dreaded enemy, you might know
comes right on time,
and once again the hope for that little miracle is gone
for at least another month or so.

Dianne Fossett 4/1/03
Used with permission

CHAPTER 2—ESTABLISHING FAITH THROUGH TRIALS

Filling the "Void"

If you're like me, you just want to feel normal again. You probably just want to feel good again, like there's no cloud hanging over your shoulders. To make myself feel better, I would fill the "void" with things that made me feel good. I would get my hair and nails done; pretty clothes lined my closet – and that's okay. However, I started making myself feel good in unhealthy ways too.

One of the extreme ways was exalting my husband to the point that he was number one in my life instead of God. Other examples of filling the void include chemical addictions such as smoking, alcohol and drugs, excessive shopping, overeating, promiscuousness… anything that gives instant gratification. When we are hurting, we numb ourselves, but the surge of joy is short lived. It's like trying to force a square block into a triangular hole.

Let me explain something very simplistically. That void is a "God-shaped hole" in your heart. Once you let God take His proper place in your heart, then and only then, will you enjoy the *"…peace of God, which transcends all understanding."*[1] The way to do this is by allowing the Lord to be the Master of your life. In doing so, he will fill your heart with His presence and His unending love and He will guard your mind with His Holy Spirit. Trusting in the Lord also allows you to experience strength, hope, and freedom… strength in your purpose for living, hope for your future and freedom from the bondage of sin.

Christy wrote an article that revealed her walk in your shoes. Read a few paragraphs she wrote about the conversation she had with her Maker; I believe it perfectly personifies the peace God intends for each of you:

"'Delight yourself in the Lord and he will give you the desires of your heart' Psalm 37:4. That scripture always sounded so simple to me – my desire was to have a baby and I reminded God of this often. Now I realize how selfishly I looked at this verse. I held onto the part that was easy and satisfied my longings, and I ignored the rest. After many months, thousands of dollars, painful medical procedures, and two miscarriages, God began to get my attention… and I began to pay attention to the entire verse.

God asked me a question that would forever change my life – one that opened my eyes to the entire psalm that meant so much to me. 'Do you love me enough?' 'Well, don't be silly, God, of course I love You enough.' 'Do you love me enough to be happy and joyful if my plan for your life does not include having a child?'

God was asking me to truly 'delight myself in Him' and let Him fill that God-sized hole in my heart that I thought was child-sized. I had to decide if I really believed all the things I said about God: He knows what's best; He wants to bless me; His timing is perfect; He loves me more than I could imagine, and so much more. I was broken at the very moment I answered 'yes.'

'Yes, God, I choose to trust You with my life, even if Your plans are different from mine. Yes, God, I choose to be joyful in all circumstances, even if I am never a mom. Yes, God, I love you enough!'

For the first time, I felt what it was like to have total peace, contentment, and joy. For the first time, God and God alone, was enough."[2]

Getting you to the point where you can say what Christy said, *"Yes, God, I choose to trust You with my life, even if Your plans are different from mine. Yes, God, I choose to be joyful in all circumstances, even if I am never a mom. Yes, God, I love you enough!"* is the mission of this book. I highly doubt you could say that right now, so keep reading with an open mind and learn the keys to healing. Learn that a "void" was placed in you with a purpose – to draw you nearer to the Lover of your Soul.

Realizing Your Sincere Motives

"The Chase" poem in the introduction of this book illustrates my encounter with infertility. I'm sure you recognize the bunny as symbolic of the baby that never came naturally. The bunny eluded me as I chased it down the trail. It skirted behind rocks and dashed quickly away. I chased in vain, yet it was worth it because I am stronger for it now. I want you to be able to feel that way some day soon.

For now, there must be something deep inside you and me to make us work so hard for the bunny. Let's take a look at what motivates *you deep down inside*.

I mentioned in my testimony that I had always wanted to be a mommy. To be truly honest with you, I don't believe my motives were to raise children just because I loved being around them. In actuality, I hadn't stopped to think about it. To me, it was a natural part of life that I just expected. When it wouldn't and then couldn't happen, I wanted it because I couldn't have it. I liken myself to a child whose toy is taken away. It's not that they want the toy so badly; they want it because it was taken from them. They cry, pout and have a fit until their tormentor returns the toy.

CHAPTER 2—ESTABLISHING FAITH THROUGH TRIALS

It's not fun admitting this for the very first time, however, I want you to stop and think about this for a moment. What are the *real* reasons you want a child so badly? You listed some in the first three questions preceding this chapter. Take some time to look back at your answers and then think about it.

For instance, in retrospect, there were two other reasons I wanted children and I am embarrassed at how selfish they were: One, I didn't want to grow old and not have a family to share memories with. Two, my husband was a self-admitted work-a-holic and I was extremely lonely. I thought the presence of children would liven up our home and fill my needs. In my naivety, I thought I could design a family and therefore, force my husband to spend time at home with us.

Does it sound like my motives were good? Not really. Fear was at the core of my desire for children. I wish I had taken the time to ponder the motivation for my intense desire. I want you to take a deep look into your heart and think about what drives you to undergo embarrassing tests and humiliating questions from your doctors. What is so important that you would subject yourself to needles and even surgery to conceive? Why are you willing to spend thousands of dollars? Of course, a baby is priceless, but there must be something deep inside that makes you yearn for a child so intensely.

Consider the following reasons I have heard from the ladies in my Bible study and witnessed by speaking to people through the years:

It's Natural:
    1. After you've been married for awhile people seem to think you're at the "age" to multiply.
    2. After experiencing marriage, the next step seems to be parenthood.
    3. You want to go through pregnancy, feel life within you, and then experience childbirth and the joy of nursing.
    4. Everyone you know has children naturally and you don't want to be left out.

Time is Running Out:
    1. You feel the pressure of society or family to give birth before you turn 40 years old.

Children are a Joy:
    1. You've always enjoyed children and want to move from babysitting, coaching or teaching to mothering.
    2. A child would remove loneliness from your life. You want a constant companion.

Family Pressure:
1. Pregnancy would cease the tormenting questions, remarks and nagging from family members or friends.
2. You want to fulfill your husband's desire for children.

Intimacy, Family Ties, or Security:
1. You grew up in a healthy family setting and you want to give that structure to a child.
2. You grew up with great morals and values that you want to pass on.
3. You feel a baby would strengthen the bond between you and your husband.
4. You want to carry on your husband's heritage.
5. Your mother and mother-in-law hound you to give them grandchildren.

Control:
1. You and your husband planned a family before your marriage and you want to stay "on schedule."

Filling the Void:
1. You feel a child will decrease the pain you feel due to an abortion in the past.

Hiding:
1. You are hiding behind the real issues in your life. Your friends and family won't notice hidden problems with addictions while they are focusing on your barrenness.

Self Expectations:
1. You've always dreamed of being a mommy and you want to see a child with your nose and daddy's ears.
2. You have been successful at everything you've done in life and the thought of "failure" to reproduce terrifies you.

Future Memories:
1. You want to share holidays and memories with a family of your own.

Now that you've considered your original answers and then read the above lists, have your answers changed? Your motivations may or may not have changed, but one thing remains the same—you need to know what is compelling you.

If you are experiencing secondary infertility, I want you to use the space below to describe your motives for wanting more children. Be truthful. Search your heart and think about your reasons. Do you just love being pregnant? Do you long to see the reaction on your husband's face when your baby emerges from your womb again? Do you feel most "only children" are usually spoiled rotten? Do you feel you are an outstanding mother and therefore you desire to give unconditional love to more children? Are you just trying to keep up with your sister-in-law? Please explain:

_____

_____

_____

Dianne's motives seem perfectly natural: *"The journey through secondary infertility is not an easy road to travel. You know exactly what you are missing and you long for another opportunity to care for and cuddle another precious little one.*

The longing makes your heart ache and your arms become limp because they can't hold another baby. You long to do some things differently because you learned valuable lessons the first time around. You want to have another chance to strive to do better."

Charlene's perspective on child-bearing seemed to change overnight. Read what led to her intense desire:

"When I married in 1993, having children was the last thing on my mind. As far as I was concerned, children were noisy, dirty, smelly, annoying inconveniences that I didn't want or need. I proclaimed these facts loudly – and often – to anyone ill-informed enough to ask me when my husband and I were going to start our family.

I was a college-educated newspaper reporter who saw no sense in spending four years and thousands of dollars in schooling only to stay home and change diapers. I was quite content being a 'family-of-two.'

However, God has a sense of humor. About five years into our marriage, I quite literally, woke up one morning in an absolute panic, I needed a baby and I needed one RIGHT NOW! My husband claims he saw subtle changes in my attitude toward children long before I had this epiphany. All I know is that I had a sudden moment of terror at the thought of dying childless and forgotten. Assuming I will outlive my husband, I didn't want my obituary to read: 'Survivors include her five cats.' (Which is odd considering I don't even have any cats.)" Charlene S. Engeron

Now, look back at questions four and five. If you do not know your husband's reasons for wanting a family with you, you need to stop and ask him. I don't intend to make things tense in your home, but communication between you and him are particularly important right now. If you have been proven to be fertile and your husband is staring sterility in the face, be especially gentle with him. His masculinity is on the line in many cases. He may be torn up inside and not sure how to handle his own disappointment. Likewise, if you desire a second or third child, consult your mate and confirm that his feelings are mutual.

Let me explain why I feel motives are so important. For instance, if passing on traits to a child are your main motivation, adoption might be a difficult alternative for you. If you are using a child to "save" your marriage, obviously you need to admit this and seek counseling immediately. Some people conceive just to please others in their lives. Do you believe this is justification to be a parent? I guess, but if you want to be *great* parents, it's not.

Cultivating Faith

As you can see by my testimony, when I was in your shoes, I grasped for peace, but I didn't really want to mess with faith. I believed in God, but I felt like I had to *make* things happen for myself. Of course, it was rough. The pain and ache I had for a child seemed relentless. It seemed as if it would never cease. I didn't understand why I had to experience weakness and vulnerability to become strong. Why couldn't I just breeze through life like most people? The answer is, if I had no problems, no worries, and everything was easy, I wouldn't need faith. I wouldn't need God. I could rely on myself and unknowingly lose out on the plans my Father in heaven had in store for me.

Unfortunately, I was foolish and stubborn and inadvertently chose to persevere on my own. Instead of looking "up" for help, I looked in the mirror. No one could relate with my feelings of emptiness... and I didn't really give God a chance.

I searched in vain for years and years for answers – the main one being "why?" As I mentioned in the previous chapter, finally in exasperation I found the answer in these verses:

> *"Consider it pure joy, my brothers, whenever you face trials of many kinds, because you know that the testing of your faith develops perseverance. Perseverance must finish its work so that you may be mature and complete, not lacking anything."*
> **James 1:2-4**

These verses are like keys. Once I used the "keys," I understood that God wasn't picking on me or punishing me. He's a loving God who has compassion for sinners. I could finally see these verses as promises for a complete life. Through persevering in faith, I would not lack anything. It was years later that I comprehended that these verses weren't promising me a baby, they were promising me a *full life God's way*—a life that may or may not include motherhood. I implore you to think about what I am saying here and not waste as much time as I did.

You would be wise to memorize James 1:2-4. Hold these verses dear to your heart as a promise. Place them somewhere you will read often and hold tight to them during the difficult times. Allow me to break them down:

"Consider it pure joy"—Joy? Yes joy. Perhaps you should be grateful your trial isn't something worse. Stop, look around, and think of what could be worse— there are many things! God gave you this trial because He knew in His infinite wisdom that you could handle this and not something else at this time in your life. In fact, it's a promise.

Look at 1 Corinthians 10:13— *"...And God is faithful; he will not let you be tempted beyond what you can bear. But when you are tempted, he will also provide a way out so that you can stand up under it."* I acknowledge that this is hard to accept, but think about it. I guarantee a day will come along when you will look back and it will make sense to you.

Pastor Tom Mercer of High Desert Church in Victorville, CA[3] spoke on this passage several years ago. He said, *"One of the basic building blocks of joy is the ability to wait. The only way God can teach us to wait is through difficult circumstances."* He continued, *"This way we keep the 'big picture' in mind."*

"Whenever you face trials of many kinds"—Pastor Mercer also said that *"We should anticipate problems."* James didn't say *"if"* you face trials, he said *"when"* you face trials, and he said they would be *"trials of many kinds."* Peter even went further in 1 Peter 4:12 by saying, *"Dear friends, do not be surprised at the painful trial you are suffering, as though something strange were happening to you."*

"Perseverance must finish its work so that you may be mature and complete, not lacking anything"—I believe this means that once you've gone through a difficulty, you come out on the other side stronger and as a more mature Christian. You will *"not be lacking anything,"* however, that may mean giving birth, fostering or adopting, or nurturing through other avenues.

All in all, everyone has problems and God shows his love by the trials He gives us. Some are physical; others are emotional, psychological or spiritual. Your trial is infertility and the faster you learn to accept it as a potential source of joy, the better off you will be. You have the keys at your disposal, leave the dark, gloomy room you are in and unlock the door to a life of faith, joy and peace.

Trials "Grow You Up" in Faith

"Blessed is the man [or woman] who perseveres under trial, because when [she] has stood the test, [she] will receive the crown of life that God has promised to those who love him."
James 1:12

I doubt anyone likes tests. Pop quizzes are the worst in my opinion. However, God's testing is different. Through the testing of your faith, you mature in your spiritual walk. God isn't setting you up for a fall, He's "growing you up" in faith and assurance.

Get your Bible out again and read 2 Peter 1:2-8. These verses basically say that to experience peace, you need to get to know God better. This takes action. Seven actions to be exact—they are:

Growing in faith
Choosing obedience
Gaining knowledge from God's Word
Exhibiting self control
Molding perseverance
Practicing humility
Gracing others with love (which comes with ultimate maturity).

These actions do not come naturally, they require work and trust. Ask God and trust Him to keep you from sin and help you live out these actions in your life. When you feel like giving up, go back and re-read these verses. Here's a great example of a woman named Christine who wanted to give up, but she relied on faith instead. This is part of a letter she wrote to me several years ago:

"I just don't know what to do. I'm either at the point of acceptance or I'm ready to give up. John and I have done everything we can to make the best

decisions and follow all the right steps in trying to have a baby. I just can't do it anymore. We are moving to a different state soon and I have to concentrate on that. I just have come to a point where faith now has to lead me. I just have to believe God would not let that happen again [ectopic pregnancy].

I have heard over and over again that God chooses to bless everyone with different gifts, but not everyone is given the same gifts. We must not be discontented with our own gifts. God has given me a wonderful family, a wonderful husband and beautiful marriage, our health, and a good career. I just have to somehow find the strength to focus on those gifts.

I can't be in control anymore. It is too hard and so hard on my body, as you very well know. After, being pregnant I just am not ready for adoption. This all may change, but this is how I have come to peace for now. I am struggling so much, but I have been praying and listening. I think God is trying to tell me that this is not the time, and I have to go on. Just as you have told me, God will not let anything happen that we can't handle in our lives, and this just is not the time."

Christine and her husband relocated, got settled in their new home, accepted very good jobs, found a good infertility specialist, continued their faith in God's timing, and they were just recently blessed with a precious baby boy.

You see, once you trust in the Lord completely, you are "fruitful," meaning others can see your faith through the way you live. God is able to "use you" to have an impact on other people's lives and hopefully their spirituality as well.

Now go back to 2 Peter 1 and read verse nine and read what happens when you don't take "faith actions." Choose wisely.

Fear Steals Your Joy

As life bustles around you in the form of baby strollers, television commercials selling diapers and formula, and you long to wear maternity clothes and shop in the children's department, it is very easy to fall into a negative pattern of fear. It seems natural that when the joy you desire is replaced with longing and despair, fear often sets in.

I believe this is because fear comes from Satan and faith comes from God. How can fear and faith exist in the same heart at the same time? The answer is: they can't. They can't because Satan and God can't cohabitate in the same heart either. I didn't realize I was afraid because I took my eyes off God and behaved the way the enemy wanted me to, by focusing on what I didn't have.

How about you? Are you feeling fearful? Take the time to look at the fears you listed on question 10. Go to God and ask Him to take them from you. Trust me, His shoulders are broad enough to bear them. In fact, the circumstances that are causing you fear may be the same circumstances that increase your faith and lead you to the peace that currently seems so illusive. Your joy will return when you give God your whole heart, not just pieces of it.

Peace is a "Heart Thing"

You may be too wrapped up in *"the chase"* to realize you are missing peace—I know I was. Peace equals clarity, and for me, clarity had been replaced with confusion, restlessness and impatience. My "plan" wasn't working. Because my marriage was rocky and I lacked the support of my helpmate, I faced sheer frustration in the knowledge that I couldn't make a baby on my own. Even if he had been interested in creating a family, my husband's work schedule and traveling did not correlate with my ovulation schedule. I couldn't adopt by myself. And, to make matters worse, I had no say in the matter. In my green eyes, my future looked bleak and further loneliness stared me in the face. I could totally relate with Rachel who said, *"Give me children or I'll die"* in Genesis 30:1 (NLT).

Jeremiah 29:11-13 helped me exchange my out-of-control quest for peace: *"For I know the plans I have for you," declares the Lord, "plans to prosper you and not to harm you, plans to give you hope and a future. Then you will call upon me and come and pray to me, and I will listen to you. You will seek me and find me when you seek me with all your heart."* When you seek after God with your heart, then He can bless you with His plans for you. Perhaps that's why Jesus said, *"Love the Lord your God with ALL your HEART and with all your soul and with all your mind,"* in Matthew 22:37.

Now picture a woman who loves her child with all her heart, that's a good thing right? Yes, to an extent. Some women give their hearts to their children and there's little or no heart left for their husband, nor God. Some of us give our hearts to our husband and inadvertently leave God with our leftover love. I know you're probably thinking, *"I won't do that AFTER God grants me a baby!"* Believe me, it's incredibly easy to do. Have you ever stopped to think that God knows you so well that He is jealous for all of your heart? Think about it.

Now, let's talk more about peace. *"Peace I leave with you; my peace I give you, I do not give to you as the world gives. Do not let your hearts be troubled and do not be afraid,"* is a promise from Jesus Christ himself in John 14:27.

CHAPTER 2—ESTABLISHING FAITH THROUGH TRIALS

Where do you search for peace? Do you go to the world looking for it in the form of people, places, substances, or materialism? Do you go to the Bible looking for it? Do you lock yourself in your home and rely on your mate for it? To experience the *"peace of God, which transcends all understanding"* (Philippians 4:7), give your heart to your Savior —*all* of your heart!

"For the eyes of the LORD range throughout the earth to strengthen those whose hearts are fully committed to him," **2 Chronicles 16:9.**

Chapter 3-Developing a Relationship with Christ

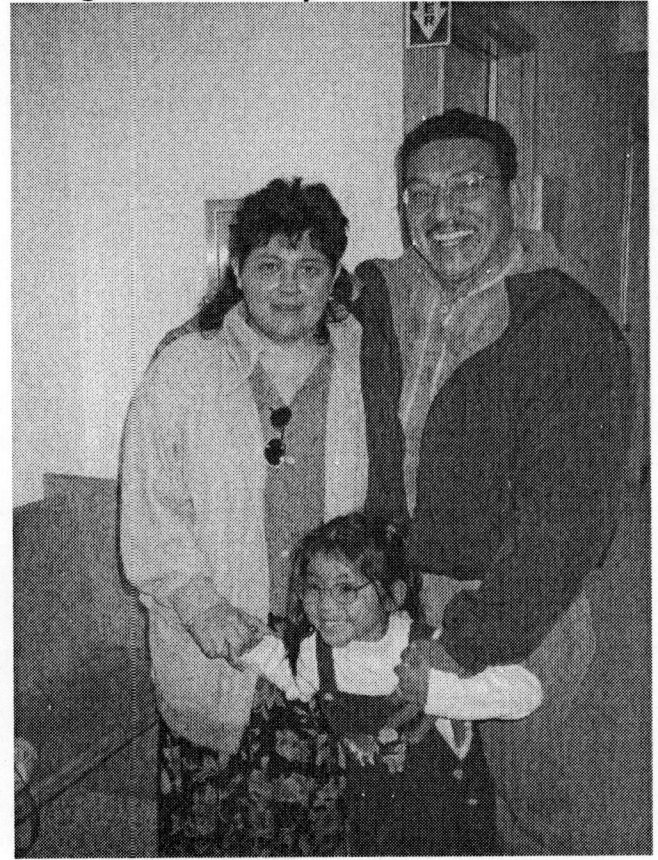

Irene, Froilan and Monica

-Feeling Empty
    Addressing Loneliness
    You are Not Alone
-Getting to Know Christ
    Through Your Suffering, Bring Honor to God
    Obtaining "Oneness" with God

Chapter 3-Developing a Relationship with Christ

1. How would you rate your relationship with God/Jesus/Holy Spirit? Please circle one:
   a) Seeking the One true God
   b) Believe in God, but not Jesus
   c) New Christian
   d) Mature Christian
   e) Agnostic
   f) Aethiest

2. If you consider yourself a Christian, describe the moment you gave Jesus Christ control of your life. Can you name the date or circumstances? Explain:

_____

_____

_____

3. If you are a non-believer, what do you believe a relationship with Christ would involve? Please explain:

_____

_____

_____

4. "Oneness" with God is when He is your Owner *and* Master. Occasionally people accept God as their Father/Owner, however someone or something else masters them (such as sin). List one big thing in your life that causes you to sin? (Pride? Self-pity? Anger? Addictions? Disobedience to God in general? A person? Selfish desires?)

_____

_____

_____

5. What are the little, everyday things that seem to constantly make you sin? (Lying? Gossiping? Envying others? Fear? Negative thoughts? Unforgiveness?)

_____

_____

_____

6. Do you like to be alone when you are struggling with an issue? Yes or No? If not, how do you handle difficulties? (Talking to a friend? Lots of friends? Your mother? Your husband? God?)

_____

_____

_____

CHAPTER 3—DEVELOPING A RELATIONSHIP WITH CHRIST

7. Has loneliness been a problem for you? Yes or No? Do you run to seclusion or do you seek reassurance from others? Explain:

_____

_____

_____

8. Are you aware that Jesus regularly spent quiet time alone with God while He walked this earth? Yes or No?

9. List three things that are important to you: (Examples: Family, husband, money, security, status, God, etc.)
    1. _____ 2. _____
    3. _____

10. List three areas you put your time, money and energy into: (Examples: Infertility testing, entertainment, recreation, hobbies, home interior, church, etc.)
    1. _____ 2. _____
    3. _____

11. Can you think of a barren woman in the Bible? Yes or No? If so, please name her/them:

_____

_____

_____

Recommended Reading:

Genesis 1:27   Psalms 62:1-2, 139
Jeremiah 9:23-24   Matthew 7:21-23, 14:13 and 23, 15:8-9
Mark 16:9-20   John 14:6 and 15-18, 17:3

Romans 6:23
Galatians 3:20
Colossians 3:1-11
2 Peter 1:2-9
Revelation 3:14-22

1 Corinthians 2:9
Ephesians 1:5
Hebrews 11:6
1 John 4:16

Look up these verses and fill in the blanks:

John 3:16: *"For God so* _____ *the world that he gave his only Son, so that everyone who*_____ *in him will not perish but have eternal life."*

Hebrews 13:5b: *"... because God has said, 'Never will I*_____*you; never will I*_____ *you.'"*

"Why me?"
Answer #2—A barren womb is designed to strengthen your relationship with your Father above and introduce you to the saving power of His Son, Jesus Christ.

Chapter 3—Hannah's Story

My name is Hannah. I'm sort of known for my long bout with infertility. It was an agonizing journey of faith; let me explain. During my era, it was customary for men in the land of Canaan to have more than one wife. This allowed them to produce larger numbers of offspring to help in their work and continue their lineage.

To me, bearing children was my duty. Being barren made me feel like a failure, mainly because my husband's other wife, Peninnah, had children. It was incredibly difficult living in the same home with her. She continually ridiculed me and loneliness sent me into fits of depression. I cried so hard I couldn't even eat.

Thankfully Elkanah (my husband) loved me and didn't divorce me, yet I sensed his embarrassment. One night he tried to make me feel better by saying 'Why make such a fuss over having no children? Isn't having me better than having ten sons?' I couldn't believe it! Why couldn't he see my misery? How could he be so self-centered and inconsiderate?

My saving grace was my faith in the Lord. He was my refuge and my strength. One night after supper I went to the Tabernacle in Shiloh and prayed to my God. He was always there for me – I knew He heard my prayers. I cried bitterly as I prayed and I made this vow to Him: 'O Lord of heaven, if you will look down upon my sorrow and answer my prayer and give me a son, then I will give him back to you, and he'll by yours for his entire lifetime, and his hair shall never be cut.'

I hadn't realized it, but Eli the Priest was watching me, and he misunderstood my mouth moving as I prayed through my tears and he accused me of being drunk. I told him, 'Oh, no, sir! I'm not drunk. But I am very sad and I was pouring my heart out to the Lord.' He made my day by replying, 'In that case, cheer up! May the Lord of Israel grant you your petition, whatever it is!'

I was finally happy again and when we returned to our home in Ramah, I became pregnant! I was so grateful I named my son Samuel, which means 'asked of God.'[1]

We can learn great lessons from Hannah– one that I want to point out is her faithfulness. She waited so long for her son and instead of selfishly clinging to him; she kept her word and returned him to the Lord. Because of his mother's obedience, God was able to shape Hannah's son, Samuel, from the start. He was a true servant of God and because he spent his childhood assisting Eli in the Temple, God was able to direct him to great responsibilities including priest, prophet, counselor and judge.

> *"I am the woman who stood here that time praying to the Lord!*
> *I asked him to give me this child, and he has given me my request;*
> *and now I am giving him to the Lord for as long as he lives."*
> **1 Samuel 1:26-28 (NLT)**

Feeling Empty

Hannah must have been so lonely and misunderstood. Not only was she sharing her husband with another woman, she was a social outcast for being barren, her husband offered her little support, and even a priest misunderstood her. I really admire this woman – instead of getting mad or getting even, she prayed to the Lord and trusted *him* to "complete her."

The Living Bible makes these points about Hannah: *"Earlier Hannah had been discouraged to the point of being physically sick and unable to eat. Here she returns home well and happy. The change in her attitude may be attributed to three factors: 1) her honest prayer to God (verse 1:11 in 1 Samuel 1:23), 2) her resolve to leave the problem with God (1:18), and 3) the encouragement she received from Eli, the priest.*

Although we are not in a position to barter with God, he may still choose to answer a prayer, which has an attached promise. When you pray, ask yourself, 'Will I follow through on any promises I make to God if he grants my request?' It is dishonest and dangerous to ignore a promise, especially to God."[2]

Please note that Hannah kept her promise and took her three-year-old son back to the Tabernacle in Shiloh. She left him with Eli to serve God in the Tabernacle (see verses 1:27-28). Giving up the son she begged God for must have been agonizing, yet she rejoiced. Joy replaced her sorrow. Her prayer of thanks can be found in 1 Samuel 2:1-10.

Hannah's Story mentions that in her day it was permissible for a man to divorce his wife on grounds of barrenness. Evidently the same is true these days; read how Gail's first marriage ended due to her inability to bear children:

"I remember telling my husband one day that I was not happy and that something was missing in my life (now I know it was Jesus Christ). My husband's response was: 'Do you think I'm happy being with a wife who can't have children?' I felt so hurt. How much lower could I go when I was already feeling like such a failure as a woman?

We eventually divorced. The pressures of infertility were too much to bear. I remember asking God: 'Will I ever be able to find a man who will love me even though I can not have children?' Two years later, my second husband to be came into my life. It was a long distance relationship for four months. I remember asking him on the phone, 'Are you fine with the fact that I may never have children?' He seemed to be, but I don't think he quite comprehended what that really meant. One year into our marriage, we both gave our lives over to the Lord and got baptized by the Holy Spirit. This was the big turning point in our lives – we now had someone to put our trust in and depend on to make this infertility issue more bearable," Gail recollects.

Gail was afraid to go through further testing because of the emotional roller coaster she went through with her first husband. A Bible study that she worked on titled "Experiencing God: Knowing and Doing the Will of God" by Henry T. Blackaby and Claude V. King made her realize that she and her husband needed to work on their marriage. *"I felt God was telling us to learn how to*

CHAPTER 3—DEVELOPING A RELATIONSHIP WITH CHRIST

understand each other and to communicate better," she said.

While Gail and her husband, Tim, put off testing to work on their marriage, things even got rockier when a female foreign exchange student moved in with them. Gail began to feel jealous of the attention her husband gave this girl, but read how Gail relied on Jesus this time: *"There I was, four years into my second marriage and it was falling apart. I kept thinking, not again! What is wrong with me? I can't even hold my marriage together. I was depressed and miserable. Then I remembered that God was in control and I needed to rest in Him. I'm so thankful I had God in my life this time. I would never have survived another day without Him there. I found a letter that helped me during my deepest depression. It reads:*

'My Dear Lost Sheep, You ask me where I am. My child, I am with you and I always will be. You are weak, but in Me, you are strong. I know what you are going through, for I am going through it with you. I will direct you in my path of righteousness. My child, I love you and I will never forsake you, for you are truly mine. Don't compare yourself to others. Know Me and Trust Me. I am pleased with you. I know that the desire of your heart is to show others your love for me. I am working in your life so that you will grow even more. Let Me be the courage you need to stand. Love, God'

After reading that letter, getting counseling from a pastor, and finding a different host home for the exchange student, I made it through the storm. God was faithful. He turned a bad situation into something wonderful. Our marriage is stronger because of this struggle in our lives," reported Gail.

God is always faithful to His "dear sheep" (mankind). Look at the last part of *"The Chase,"* it reads: *"Raise baby to sky. Shout 'thank you!' to the heavens. 'God is good! God is love!' Baby vanishes. Arms still in the air. Cry out 'God is peace!'"* The interpretation is that only God can fill the "empty void" in your life. By *allowing* yourself to feel *complete* as a family of two (or three or four if you have children) you accept His gift of peace.

Furthermore, children belong to God. If you are blessed with a child, you will eventually have to let them go. However, they were never yours to begin with, so in actuality, you are borrowing them for a season. If you are *not* blessed with a child, I promise that if you allow God to grant you with peace to move on as a complete family, He will!

I'll be brutally honest; continuing to feel empty is a choice. A better choice is choosing to fill your life with the opposite of emptiness, which is fullness. The *American Heritage Dictionary* defines fullness as: *"Complete, with nothing lacking."*[3]

Addressing Loneliness

Unfortunately, most barren women experience the loneliness Hannah felt. It feels like you're sinking in quicksand. Even if you suspect your husband may be sterile, I surmise your loneliness is great because you can't completely relate with his feelings of lack of performance.

Mothers with secondary infertility often feel alone because people in their world accuse them of being ungrateful for what they've got. The women I have talked with long for another child as much as any of us, however, they have no place to share their feelings without sounding like they are complaining or unappreciative of the child(ren) they've been blessed with. Consequently, these ladies usually keep their desire for more children secret.

Janet remembers how she felt several years ago: *"It's hard to deal with secondary infertility because you are subjected to the never-ending children's birthday parties, preschool activities and school functions where parents are either pregnant, announcing another pregnancy or letting you know they are trying for another one this month. I would usually be asked, 'So, when are you going to give Jake a little brother or sister?'*

I didn't want to explain why it wasn't happening yet I thought everyone was wondering if I couldn't handle another one or if I didn't enjoy being a mother. It was so uncomfortable that I didn't want to attend these functions. However, I wasn't fair to make my son miss them just because I was hurting—I was basically stuck in situations I couldn't avoid.

When people eventually found out I was having a hard time getting pregnant they usually said, 'You should just be thankful you already have a child.' Jake's own comments broke my heart; his sweet, little face would look at me, and he'd ask 'Why don't I have a brother or sister? Can I have one? All my friends and cousins have them.' We would go to the mall and he would ask for a penny to throw into the fountain to make a wish. Every time he threw the penny in, he would close his eyes real tight and wish for a baby brother or sister.

The cruelest comments came from my own mouth: 'maybe I am a horrible mother and God sees me as unfit and that is why he hasn't blessed me with another child. What am I doing wrong? Am I not attractive enough to my husband to make a baby? It's a confusing, lonely time," Janet recalled.

Everyone experiences loneliness at some point in his or her lives; it can be all-consuming if you let it. When you are experiencing it, it feels like no one else in the world knows how you feel—wrong. Allow me to paint a surprising,

CHAPTER 3—DEVELOPING A RELATIONSHIP WITH CHRIST

personification of loneliness. Picture a church in your mind. You might envision stained glass windows, an altar and velvet padded pews, or you might even picture a gymnasium complete with a stage and podium, a cross, and folding chairs.

In the front row sits Amy, a 17-year-old girl dressed in a baggy, teal-colored dress. Her head hangs low as she sits next to her mother. Feeling ashamed as she sits in the presence of the Lord, these thoughts leave her feeling light headed: *I can't believe I am pregnant – I was only with Joey once! How do I tell him? How do I tell my parents? They'll be so disappointed in me! I'm sitting here with a baby in my womb and yet I feel so alone.*

Behind the young girl sits a professionally dressed couple. The woman, probably in her early 30's, looks distressed as she stares at Amy and ponders these thoughts: *I was so naïve when I was that girl's age. I believed all the nursery rhymes I sang about marriage and baby carriages in the same sentence. She's young and unaware of the big problems life throws at us—she's probably thinking about football games and high school dances, while I sit here feeling so disappointed and desperate. No one in my world understands the agony I experience as I go from one fertility expert to the next. Why won't you bless me with just one child Lord? I'm only asking for one!*

Several rows back sits a couple with their 18-month-old baby girl all dressed in lace. Their adoration for her is quite evident as they stare at her almost oblivious to the service going on around them. They look so happy, yet the mother, Jenna, has thoughts no one else knows about. She closes her eyes and prays to the Lord: *Oh God, Samantha means everything to me. Why can't I conceive again? Am I doing something wrong in my life or in my marriage? Am I wrong to think I'm a good mother? Are you keeping a child from me for some reason? Now that my body shape has changed somewhat, is Brian not attracted to my anymore? He seems so happy to be a father, yet our love life is lacking. Please talk to me God – I need you to talk to me!*

Meanwhile, Brian winks at Jenna, coos at his daughter and while the church members probably think he's got the world by the tail his private thoughts are filled with loneliness too. *Jesus,* he prays. *You know I love you and I thank you for answering our prayers for a baby, but I am really struggling. I never want to seem ungrateful for Samantha, but I miss my wife Lord! She's so dedicated to the baby's needs that she's forgotten about my needs. All she talks about is having another child. She doesn't go to her Bible study anymore or even take the time to pray with me. I'm ashamed for feeling jealous of my own daughter, however, I really need your help!*

Captured in their own thoughts, Jenna and Brian are unaware of the quiet tears Amanda sheds as she sits two seats back. *Should I get up and leave?* She wonders. *Here people surround me and I am so lonely. I might as well go home. I'm too angry to praise you Lord and I can't stay here and watch Jenna and Brian with Samantha for one more minute. They are so lucky! Why did you choose to give Samantha to them instead of Carlos and me? Why did you take our baby before we even got to see her? I hurt so bad Jesus. I don't think I'll ever experience happiness or peace again.*

Closer to the back of the church hides Laura, a mother of three rambunctious children. *Hopefully no one will see me back here. I look like a mess*, she thinks. *Now that little Jimmy has come along I don't have time for myself anymore*, she complains to herself. *Oh, there's Jenna and Brian up there. Wow, it must be nice only having one kid – they've got it so easy! I can't believe Jenna's been whining about not getting pregnant again. She should just leave well enough alone.*

Oh, and there's Amanda. I bet she's still crying over her miscarriage. It's been three months now – for heaven's sake she needs to get over it. I know; I'll let her borrow my little Jimmy – that'll shut her up! She just doesn't realize how rough motherhood really is. I can't even go to the bathroom alone anymore or have adult conversations. Sometimes I just wish I had my old life back.

When you experience "the darkness" of a trial, sometimes you are so consumed that you don't even realize other people are suffering with their own trials. Like I said, loneliness can be all-consuming *if you let it,* so don't let it be!

First of all, find encouragement in the knowledge that you are NOT alone. According to *Stepping Stones*[4] newsletter, a publication of Bethany Christian Services that offers Christian support to couples facing infertility and pregnancy loss: *"One in 10 couples in their 20's will experience a significant infertility problem. For couples in their 30's, the ratio rises to one in six couples. And for couples seeking to have children in their 40's statistics indicate that one in four will experience infertility."*

Stop and think about those numbers, that's a lot of lonely people who need each other! Reach out to other ladies through support groups and carefully chosen online chat rooms, and consider subscribing to publications that offer encouragement and helpful articles.

Second, notice that God gives you periods in your life when you feel like you are "walking through the desert" so to speak. This is a lonely time when

CHAPTER 3—DEVELOPING A RELATIONSHIP WITH CHRIST

no one seems able to relate to you. You might equate yourself to dry tumbleweeds that stumble around the desert alone, with no purpose. I believe God gives you these times to shake you up and wake you up. He can use loneliness to draw you closer to Him.

Let me remind you that Jesus went off by himself often for quiet times with His Father. In His human form, He needed to be re-energized just like we do. He needed quiet so that He could hear with both ears just like we do. For instance, after John the Baptist's death, Jesus went off in a boat to a remote area to be alone with God, (Matthew 14:13).[5] The crowds followed Him and after taking pity on them he healed their sick and multiplied the five loaves of bread and two fish to feed 5,000 people.

Afterward, in Matthew 14:23[6] he tried once gain to retreat up into the hills to pray. Other examples are given, but my point is that He sought out personal time with God. He made it a priority and it is my opinion that He was setting a great example for us.

Look at Luke 4:42—*"At daybreak Jesus went out to a solitary place."* Once again, I believe He was showing us that even when life is really busy (remember, people were seeking Him out to heal them and perform miracles and witness to them, so He knew "busy"), we must make it a priority to get up and spend time with God first thing in the morning before the day gets too crazy.

Third, we are never alone. Jesus had to die on the cross as a ransom for our sins, and He had to die so that the Holy Spirit could reside in the hearts of those who trust Him as their Savior. As a mere mortal, He could only be in one place at a time, of course, after His ascension into heaven He was omnipresent.

He said, *"If you love me, you will obey what I command. And I will ask the Father, and he will give you another Counselor to be with you forever – the Spirit of truth,"* (John 14:15-16.) Some Bible versions call the Holy Spirit the Comforter. I like that – I need that. How about you? God sends the Comforter to direct us down the right paths and help us make good decisions. We, on the other hand, have to be responsible enough to seek out that guidance and then listen well.

Even though we are not alone, Jesus shows us that the alone-times we experience during infertility can be used to benefit our trust in Him. It causes us to pursue Him. It opens our eyes and by refocusing our thoughts, it eventually strengthens our faith in Him.

You are Not Alone

In the early stages of my struggle with infertility, I couldn't find anyone else to share this burden with. I felt like a leper—off by myself, contaminated and misunderstood. Later, after I found a few resources to share in, I began to believe that those of us chosen to undergo this affliction are really good at keeping secrets. As far as I knew, infertility was fairly unheard of and therefore, it seemed like resources and support groups were non-existent.

Thankfully things have changed over time. For instance, I am happy to include a list of resources, books and support groups in Appendix A in the back of this book. Please take advantage of them. Also, I was greatly surprised when I read the statistics in the following article. Here are two excepts from *"A Change in Flight"* by Lauren Spurr that was printed in the Oct./Nov. 2002 issue of *Stepping Stones* newsletter:

"Although you may often feel like you're on an island, separated from those happy, carpooling, troop-leading, soccer-coaching, cookie-baking mommies, the facts state otherwise. In 2000, the World Health Organization estimated that approximately eight to ten percent of couples experience some form of infertility.

What I can offer you, beyond startling statistics and the promise of God's protection, is this: He will not forsake you or leave you.[7] He does not expect you to try to 'handle' this journey on your own. He greatly desires you to NEED Him. As you commune with Him, you will find peace. Though your questions may go unanswered, and your pain may never completely cease, your Heavenly Father is a sovereign God who rules and reigns over your life. Read His Word and trust in His promises."

Finally, you are not alone once you accept Jesus as your Savior because He will reside in your heart forever. This is God living within you—you will literally never be alone again, unless you choose to live your life defying His existence or His guidance, wisdom and direction.

Getting to Know Christ

The "i" word rocked my world. It truly had an impact on my spirituality. Sometimes in my alone times, I would be so worked up that it was like a volcano stirred my insides and erupted out of my mouth. Screaming, wailing, profanity, and sheer uncontrollable hurt would hurl from my being until I lay curled up in

CHAPTER 3—DEVELOPING A RELATIONSHIP WITH CHRIST

a ball in a lonesome corner. Often I felt like hiding from God so I didn't have to feel the guilt of my outbursts. Other times, as I lay on the floor, it was like I could feel Him comforting me and soothing me. I could somehow imagine His strong arms wrapped around me as He whispered, *It's alright my child. I forgive you! I am here for you during this difficult season.*

If I haven't said it enough times, let me reiterate, He is always with you. I love Psalm 139:1-12 where King David says, *"O LORD, you have searched me and you know me. You know when I sit and when I rise; you perceive my thoughts from afar. You discern my going out and my lying down; you are familiar with all my ways. Before a word is on my tongue you know it completely, O LORD. You hem me in behind and before; you have laid your hand upon me. Such knowledge is too wonderful for me, too lofty for me to attain.*

Where can I go from your Spirit? Where can I flee from your presence? If I go to the heavens, you are there; if I make my bed in the depths, you are there. If I rise on the wings of the dawn, if I settle on the far side of the sea, even there your hand will guide me; your right hand will hold me fast. If I say, 'Surely the darkness will hide me and the light become night around me,' even the darkness will not be dark to you; the night will shine like the day, for darkness is as light to you.'"

Isn't it reassuring that someone really cares? I know the people in your life care, but they are not with you 24 hours a day, seven days a week. He is. His Word says in many places that He waits for you to call upon Him because He desires a relationship with you. (See Jeremiah 29:11-14.)

Here's more proof. Look at Matthew 7:22: *"Many will say to me on that day, 'Lord, Lord, did we not prophesy in your name, and in your name drive out demons and perform many miracles?' Then I will tell them plainly, 'I NEVER KNEW YOU. Away from me, you evildoers!'"* That evildoer would have been me! I would have been flabbergasted if I had died 12 or more years ago, met the Lord and said, *"I was a good girl. I went to church every Sunday and to confession once a month. I never killed any one and I tried to be kind,"* only to be told that, *"He never knew me!"*

The truth is, I knew *about* the King of Kings through a lifetime of rituals and religion, but I lacked a *relationship* with Him. In a friendship you trust someone, you confide in them, and you share your joys and sorrows with them. Why would anyone be hesitant about a friendship with her Father in heaven?

There are three things I want you to learn, because they will make this time much more bearable for you: One, God doesn't want a single person to perish

(2 Peter 3:9).[8] He says in Revelation 3:20: *"Here I am! I stand at the door and knock. If anyone hears my voice and opens the door, I will come in and eat with him, and he with me."* This is another reference to relationship. Think about it, when you want to get to know someone better, what do you do? Most people dine together so they can talk and become better acquainted.

If God has been "knocking on the door of your heart" and you have not responded to Him, now is the time. To accept Christ as your Savior means giving the steering wheel of your life to Him and sitting back to let Him drive. He says in John 10:10[9] that He wants to give you abundant life. Since He made you, He has a plan for your life. In fact, 1 Corinthians 2:9 states that his plan is better than anything you could dream of: *"No eye has seen, no ear has heard, no mind has conceived what God has prepared for those who love Him."*

You don't need to go anywhere, have a big ceremony or say anything fancy, just look up to the heavens or get on your knees and repeat these words with the utmost sincerity of your heart and Jesus Christ will save you from eternal death: *"Lord, please forgive me of my sins. I'm tired of doing it my way and I want you to take over and be my Lord and Savior. Please come into my life and show me how you want me to live. Amen."*

If you prayed that prayer, you are now a follower of Christ! This is a day to celebrate and one you'll never forget. Instead of just existing, now you will truly live. Call someone whom you know has been praying for your salvation and celebrate with him or her!

I'm not saying everything will be easy and you'll never experience trials again, on the contrary, but now the Holy Spirit resides in your heart and He will aid you in making good decisions and He will direct you when good verses evil. However, you must listen and obey. It would be very wise to find a Bible-based church that you feel comfortable with. The reason for this is to allow your self worship-time, Bible explanations and fellowship with other Christians.

It would also behoove you to find a Bible study group. I learned so much that reading the Bible became fun. I learned how to pray. I learned how to trust God. Faith in myself was replaced with faith in God's plan for my life. I would love that for you!

Two, reading God's Word daily will make a tremendous impact. People often complain that life is rough and there's no "owner's manual" to give guidance. Not true! God in His loving grace entrusted us with complete instructions on how to live life to the fullest. We, in turn, must make the time

CHAPTER 3—DEVELOPING A RELATIONSHIP WITH CHRIST

to read it. I find it interesting how easily I can get out of the habit of reading daily, yet I *make time* for things of lesser value such as watching television, spending two hours eating at a restaurant, going out for coffee, etc. If you find yourself in the same boat, condition yourself to get back on track.

Three, continuous prayer will enhance your relationship with God immensely. As I mentioned, I was a "religious" person for 29 years, but at the age of 30, a group of ladies in my Bible study made me realize through Matthew 15:8-9[10] and Colossians 2:20-23[11] that I possessed "head knowledge" of Jesus through legalistic religion, not a "heart relationship" with Christ. Consequently, I thought I could only pray for the "big things" and I wasn't to bother the King with "trivial" issues. Now I realize that by trusting Him with every element of my life I demonstrate faith.

If you have given your life to Jesus in the past and you have walked away from that friendship, He's waiting to hear from you too. Simply humble yourself and tell Him you miss Him and you want Him controlling your life again. He'll forgive you and welcome you back just like the example of the prodigal son in Luke 15:24.[12]

On the other hand, if you have known Jesus for a long time and you are experiencing a plateau in your spirituality or a distance between you and God, perhaps He's using this trial to strengthen your relationship with Him or make you aware of a missing link in your friendship with Him. Look at the following checklist and see what the problem might be:

Are you praying daily?
Are you reading God's Word daily?
Do you have unconfessed sin in your life?

Only you know the answers to these questions. If you need to take care of business, then do it! The truly compassionate Prince of Peace gives you salvation, prayer, the Bible, and grace—what more could you ask for?

Desires

Desires are longings of the heart.
In this season,
the desire is that of another baby.
The Bible tells us
"Delight yourself in the Lord,
and He will give you the desires of your heart."
Another baby has not been given,
This is my heart's desire.
I have delighted or so I thought.
Lord, wasn't this your promise
to give your child her heart's desire?
Did your child misunderstand?
My Lord, replied,
"No, not just now."
This desire has not come to pass,
months have gone, years have passed.
Still my heart's desire is unfulfilled,
Hope is fading, dreams are gone,
The time has come
Oh, dear Lord,
please help me understand,
Is a child a part of your sovereign and loving plan?
Lord, if not; then help your child
accept the course you charted for her.
Let truth be known in all the land,
Christ rules and reigns in the heart
of one whose desire is to
Trust in
Him.

Dianne L. Fossett, 3/20/03
Used with permission

CHAPTER 3—DEVELOPING A RELATIONSHIP WITH CHRIST

Through Your Suffering, Bring Honor to God

Infertility is so frustrating. For instance, I told my feet to walk and they did. I told my hand to pick up a spoon and it obeyed. Yet, twelve times a year I told my reproductive organs to produce an embryo and it ignored my pleas. So many of my friends set out for pregnancy and easily achieved it within months. Yet when they planned their second and third babies, their bodies ignored them as well. Our hearts and minds enter suffering mode when our bodies won't comply with our wishes.

Suffering makes you turn more and more to the only source of strength. It will refine you as gold is refined by fire. In 1 Peter 1:7 (NLT), Peter says, *"These trials are only to test your faith, to see whether or not it is strong and pure. It is being tested as fire tests gold and purifies it – and your faith is far more precious to God than mere gold; so if your faith remains strong after being tried in the test tube of fiery trials, it will bring you much praise and glory and honor on the day of his return."* Peter is basically saying that as gold is heated, impurities float to the top and can be skimmed off.

God uses adversity (or heat) to bring honor to His name, for our good, and His ultimate glory. How? By making your faith strong it shows in your "witness" to others. My friend, Irene, experienced this during her long ordeal while adopting her daughter from another country. This is how she describes her experience:

"My husband and I were trying to get pregnant; I was taking Clomid [a fertility drug], and he had surgery. We found out from the surgeon that through a childhood disease, he had become sterile. It was good to finally have an answer, however, this answer almost ripped our marriage apart. We are both from Central America where a man's masculinity is very important and it is often demonstrated by his ability to reproduce. My husband was so upset that he demanded a divorce from me. Because I am nine years younger than he is, he wanted me to marry someone else and raise a family.

Luckily, I had been invited to a women's retreat through our church and it was there that I gave my life to the Lord. When I returned home, I was in a much better frame of mind, so when he told me again of his plans to divorce, I said, 'Fine, but when people ask, you tell them the truth— that this was your idea.' He never brought it up again after that.

My husband had been against adoption, because of his machismo, but now things were different. It was shortly after my conversion that my grandmother, from El Salvador, called to say that a local woman was pregnant and needed a home for her baby. As soon as she delivered, I was on a flight and shortly after, a three-week-old baby girl was placed in my arms. My love for her was instantaneous, however, the adoption procedures weren't.

I was basically stuck in El Salvador, in my grandmother's home, for two, very long years. It took that long to go through the paperwork, fly my husband over for court procedures, obtain a visa for my daughter, and obtain a home-study from an agency near my California home. My uncle, grandmother, and other family members had been introduced to a 'new me' when I arrived in the country a new Christian. I was less volatile, more patient and I had faith in God. But the evidence of my faith was demonstrated as I went through each obstacle without becoming discouraged. Everyday I read my Bible and prayed. Often my family would comment on my faith. As usual, God took something that seemed impossible and made something wonderful out of it!"

You might not be in Irene's shoes, but you have people watching how you handle your suffering everywhere you go—at church, at work, in your neighborhood, etc. They don't know the details and they probably don't care to, however, they watch your faith. Unfortunately, some of them want you to fall on your face and curse God, because that gives them an excuse to turn from Him as well.

I believe the majority of people on this earth are searching for the One true God and *the Christ they see in you may be the only Christ they ever see.* That sounds like a lot of pressure, but remember God knows what he's doing. He knows who is watching you, and He already knows how you will react in every situation. So, rely on Him for strength, wisdom and good judgment every time you walk out your front door.

Obtaining "Oneness" With God

Oneness with God is equivalent to spiritual maturity. You become more spiritually mature 1) as you decipher what "spiritual gifts" (or special abilities) God gave you (this is covered in Chapter 10), 2) as you exercise your gifts, and 3) as you look for opportunities to use these gifts to serve God. Each member of the body of Christ is given spiritual gifts, and as we pool these gifts together, the body of Christ becomes stronger and more effective.

To me, spiritual maturity (or oneness), takes place every day of your life once you choose to live for Christ. Thankfully I learned about this a couple years into my struggle when I read an advertisement in our church bulletin for a new ladies

CHAPTER 3—DEVELOPING A RELATIONSHIP WITH CHRIST

Bible study. It must have been obvious to Cheryl, the leader of the study, that I was clueless right off the bat.

I recall the first conversation going something like this:

"Are you saved?" she asked.

"What's that?" I responded.

"Let me put it another way," she said. "If you were to die tomorrow, do you believe you would go to heaven?"

"I think so—I hope so!" I replied.

"Tell me why God should let you into heaven?" she asked.

"Because I try to be a good person and because I believe in Him," I answered.

"Do you realize that even Satan believes in Him? It takes more than belief, it takes relationship," she explained.

That conversation left me very confused because I thought the devil was down in hell waiting for all the bad people. I had a lot to learn and I am grateful for that group of ladies who patiently showed me the truth about God through His Word and diligent prayer. Every day since then I've grown in my relationship with Christ and I look forward to my spiritual growth increasing until the day I die.

Oneness with God also requires surrender. That is, putting your plans aside and relying on His plans for your life. Oneness means looking to God for your every need instead of relying on yourself. It seems obvious how oneness rewards us with peace and joy. However, do not be mislead into believing you're off the hook now. Before your conversion you were on the enemy's side; you posed no threat to him. Now you do.

He will come calling and it's critical that you are prepared. How do you prepare yourself? By reading the Bible and learning about God and His Son; by learning to listen to the coaching of the Holy Spirit; and, by praying to God and leaning on Him to help you in everything you do. Don't waste your time worrying about the evil one. Instead, invest your time in defending yourself against him. Learn how in the following chapter.

Note: If your answer to question one at the beginning of this chapter was a), b), e), or f), I hope it has changed to c)!

"Jesus answered, 'I am the way and the truth and the life. No one comes to the Father except through me.'" John 14:6

Chapter Four–Reading the Bible and Praying Daily

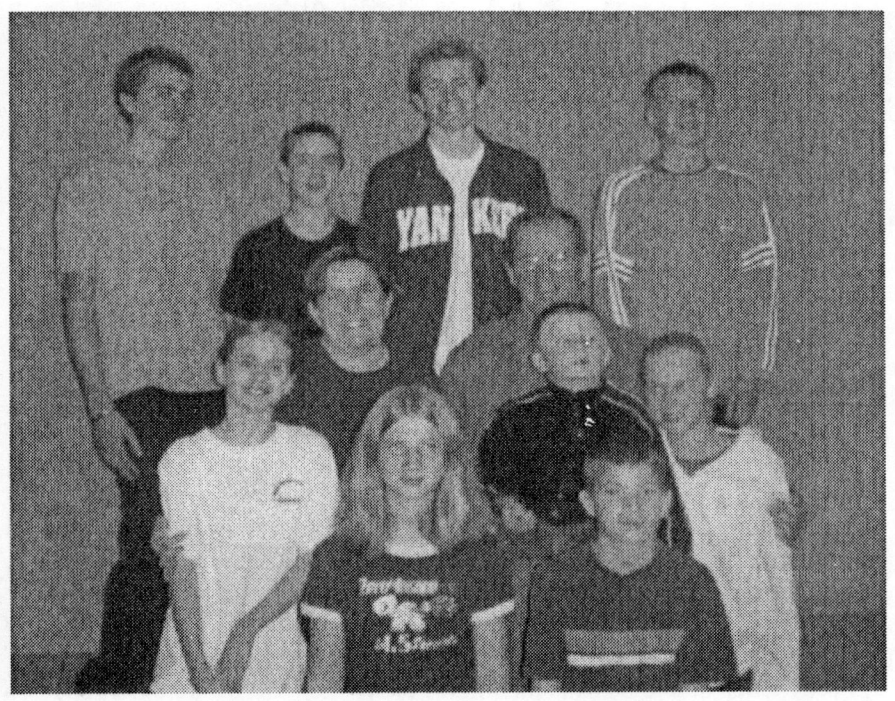

(Back row, l to r) Ben, Daniel, Sam and Paul (Middle row) Claudia and Bob (Front row) Ani, Sveta, Ivan, Steven and Marina

   -Developing a Habit of Reading God's Word Daily
        Love Letters from Your Heavenly Father
        The Bible's "Barren Society"
        "Arming" Yourself with the Word
   -Learning How to Pray
        Pray without Ceasing
        How Your Prayers are Hindered

Chapter Four–Reading the Bible and Praying Daily

1. How would you rate your Bible reading practice? (Circle one) a) I read daily. b) I read the Bible when something big is happening in my life. c) I would like to read it, but it's too difficult to understand. d) I don't read it.

2. If you *do not* read the Bible, please explain your reason(s):

_____

_____

_____

3. Some people have a difficult time believing the Bible is true. Are you aware that the Holy Spirit inspired the Bible, which was written by 40 different authors over a span of 2,000 years? To this date, nothing is contradicted; prophecy in the Old Testament is fulfilled and written about later in the New Testament. Do you believe the Bible is the Truth? Yes or No?

4. How would you rate your prayer life: a) I find myself praying all the time. b) I pray when someone asks me to. c) I pray when there's an emergency or dire situation. d) I would like to pray, but I don't know how. e) I don't pray.

5. If you do pray, what hinders your prayers the most? a) Obedience to God, b) Unconfessed sin, c) Unforgiveness (of yourself, God or others), d) Other.

6. If you do not pray, please explain your reasoning:

_____

_____

_____

7. Who do you typically put your faith in? (Yourself? Your husband? God? Fate?)

_____

_____

_____

8. Do you believe God made you perfect in His eyes? Yes or No?

9. Is having faith in God difficult for you? Yes or No? Do you believe you could live by faith and not by sight? Yes or No?

10. Do you feel God is picking on you or that He desires to strengthen your relationship with Him through this trial?

_____

_____

_____

11. Would your attitude about this trial change if you knew you only had one more day to live?

_____

_____

_____

Recommended Reading:

Joshua 1:7-8
Psalm 66:18, 119:71, 139:13-16
Mark 11:23-25

Isaiah 59:1-2
Matthew 10:29-31
Luke 6:46-49

CHAPTER 4—READING THE BIBLE AND PRAYING DAILY

John 15:7, 17:20-21
2 Corinthians 10:3-5
2 Timothy 2:19

Romans 8:14-17
Ephesians 1:11, 6:10-20
1 Peter 3:12

Look up these Verses and Fill in the Blanks:

1 Thessalonians 5:16-19 (NLT): *"Always be joyful. Always keep on _____. No matter what happens, always be thankful, for this is God's _____ for you who belong to Christ Jesus. Do not defile the Holy Spirit."*

Psalm 139:17-18 (NLT): *"How precious it is, Lord, to realize that you are thinking about me _____! I can't even count how many times a day your thoughts turn towards me. And when I awaken in the morning, you are still thinking of ____!"*

Deuteronomy 17:19-20 (NLT): *"That copy of the laws shall be his constant companion. He must read from it every day of his life so that he will learn to respect the Lord his God by _____ all of his commands. This regular _____ of God's laws will prevent him from feeling that he is better than is fellow citizens. It will also prevent him from turning away from God's laws in the slightest respect, and will ensure his having a long, good reign. His sons will then follow him upon the throne."*

"Why are you ignoring me God?"
Answer #3—A barren womb forces you to trust in the Lord, dig deep into His Word, and learn to pray for strength, obedience and wisdom daily.

Chapter 4—Rebekah's Story

I am Rebekah. My husband was Isaac, thus my father-in-law was Abraham. From what I hear, Abraham's lineage eventually led to the Savior of the world, Jesus Christ. I am so honored to be part of his ancestry! Apparently after his death on the cross, Jesus sent the Holy Spirit to live in people's hearts – that's one of the reasons he had to die. It must be so comforting for modern women to have God residing in them, comforting them, and showing them a light through dark times.

I have experienced dark times in my own life. Evidently my twin sons Esau and Jacob are featured in the Bible. Because quite a bit focuses on them, my husband, Abraham, Sarah, and other relatives, few people realize that it took me many years to get pregnant. My heart ached for a child so long after our marriage, yet my prayers were not answered.

I waited and waited. I found myself wondering if God had forgotten me. It finally got to the point where my husband pleaded with Jehovah (in Genesis 25:21), to give me a child. Then at last I conceived twins! Prayer has proven to be very important in my life in fact, it's what brought Isaac and I together.[1]

"Then I bowed my head and worshiped and blessed Jehovah, the God of my master Abraham, because he had led me along just the right path to find a girl from the family of my master's brother." **Genesis 24:48 (NLT)**

Developing a Habit of Reading God's Word Daily

People like Rebekah, who lived before Christ came to earth, didn't have the New Testament to gain wisdom and encouragement from. Thankfully, we can now consult the entire Bible during good *and* bad times. If you are having a difficult time and you find yourself pouting or feeling sorry for yourself, turn to the Bible instead of isolation. These words sound tough, but I was there and I am well aware of how easy it is to run to seclusion when you're hurting. It's the most natural thing to do, yet the most dangerous.

Let me explain. Home feels safe. You avoid blank stares from people who can't relate. You're free from admitting a problem when you're not asked *how many children do you have* nine times a day. Seclusion feels safe. If you're at home, you're not seeing newborn babies in strollers or young children feasting on chocolate ice cream.

I completely understand the logic, but trust me, this is the worst thing you can do. You are setting yourself up for attack – an assault of the blues (which is ripe territory for the enemy). You're basically making yourself a target for his fiery arrows. These arrows come in the form of physical ailments, unforeseen tragedies, marital problems, depression, and so on. We will get into staving off these attacks in the next chapter, but for now, I want to focus on how to read the Word daily.

When you are seeking comfort and peace, go to the Bible. If necessary, have them lying all over your house. When you feel the whisper of Satan telling you lies, pick that book up and read the love letters God sent to you. Yes, you. He gave you answers to every question in that "owner's manual" for life.

I had never read the Bible prior to my conversion, so I started in Genesis (the first book). It seemed logical to start "in the beginning," although I learned later that new believers should start in the New Testament, particularly in the Gospels revealed in Matthew, Mark, Luke and John. The latter became my personal favorite.

If you are new to this, I suggest you purchase or borrow a "study Bible." It paraphrases segments and breaks them down for you – a real help when you're starting out.

I also suggest that you read first thing in the morning. You'll notice that the calm you generate from God's Word will continue throughout the day. Many of my friends have mentioned how their days are very stressful and chaotic when they give God their leftover time. I agree.

> Lord, as we strive to hear
> You speak,
> As truth within Your
> Word we seek,
> Reveal to us Your holy face,
> Your love, Your will,
> Your perfect grace.

Anonymous

Love Letters from Your Heavenly Father

Our world moves at a dangerously fast pace. It seems like little kids are forced to grow up too quickly, teenagers are lost in fantasy land, newlyweds go into debt because they expect to immediately have what their parents worked years to acquire, adults who missed their childhood seek childish pleasure in unhealthy facets, and aging people chase youthfulness. It's a vicious cycle. The world seems very evil if we let it. We could easily fall into the trap of believing secular teachings such as:

- You have a right to everything you want—now go out and MAKE it happen.
- If your body is not perfect, you are less.
- You can "have it all" by stepping on others, just don't get caught.

If you listen to advertisements or look to the "world" for direction, this trial will leave you feeling less of a woman, less of a wife, and less of a Christian. Don't let it. You might be broken-hearted, but you are not defective (and neither is your husband if he is sterile). Pick up a Bible. Hold it in your hands and let me describe a scenario for a brief second.

Stop and visualize this: Picture yourself deeply in love with your husband who is far away from you for the time being. Suddenly you become aware that your beloved left a drawer full of love letters written specifically to you somewhere in the house. Wouldn't you tear that house apart looking for those letters? Wouldn't your heart race as you searched and dreamt of the sweet promises, affection and admiration that would soon be revealed on those pages?

Let me explain something. God did exactly that. He left you a volume of "love letters" in the form of the Bible. It was written by human hands, but inspired by Him through His Holy Spirit. Therefore, picture yourself finding that drawer full of love letters. Now read how much you are loved. I want you to take these verses very personally:

"For you created my inmost being; you knit me together in my mother's womb. I praise you because I am fearfully and wonderfully made; your works are wonderful, I know that full well. My frame was not hidden from you when I was made in the secret place. When I was woven together in the depths of the earth, your eyes saw my unformed body. All the days ordained for me were written in your book before one of them came to be." David, author of Psalm 139:13-16.

"Moreover, because of what Christ has done we have become gifts to God that he delights in, for as part of God's sovereign plan we were chosen from the beginning to be his, and all things happen just as he decided long ago." Ephesians 1:11 (NLT)

"The Lord is near to those who have a broken heart, and saves such as have a contrite spirit." Psalm 34:18 (NLT)

"He gives power to the tired and worn out, and strength to the weak." Isaiah 40:29

"Are not two sparrows sold for a penny? Yet not one of them will fall to the ground apart from the will of your father. And even the very hairs of your head are all numbered. So don't be afraid; you are worth more than many sparrows." Matthew 10:29-31

"Long ago, even before he made the world, God chose us to be his very own, through what Christ would do for us; he decided then to make us holy in his eyes, without a single fault—we who stand before him covered with his love." Ephesians 1:4-5 (NLT)

You can either choose to listen to the lies of this world or you can accept love and fullness from your Creator God. He says He created you perfectly, without a fault. He is so in love with you that He even counted the hairs on your head. I'm willing to bet your husband has never done that! He delights in you and considers you a gift. Several of these verses make it very clear that God had a plan for your life before you were even conceived.

Why then would you try to change the plan? Why would you try to "help" Him give you what you want instead of what He wants? Why change the plan and the timing He chose for you? First Corinthians 2:9 says that you can't even dream or fathom the plans He has for you.[2] Because He has this huge plan for you, He wants you to give up your will for your life and your timing for His will and His timing. This is called surrender.

You'll reach a point when you are ready. Believe it or not, you'll reach a point when you can say from your heart of hearts that even if His will is for you to continue life "complete" as a family of two, or a family of three, you will freely accept it without hesitation. It took me nine years to get there, and I finally did. I remember it well. A three-week-old baby girl was placed in my arms a week later. Who knows what He has in store for you, but I truly hope you will be wise and not as thick headed as I was.

The Bible's "Barren Society"

Because I was fairly unfamiliar with the Bible, it was a great relief for me to find godly women who had walked in my shoes. I needed to know that I wasn't the only one with this "dirty, little secret." There was no one in my world who could relate, so I spent time in the Bible learning about their stories. I believe my intrigue revolved more around their difficulties rather than their achievements. For instance, let's look at their struggles. They are the same obstacles we face today:

Hannah
> She struggled with low self worth because she was barren.

Rebekah
> She took initiative, but it wasn't balanced by wisdom.
> She deceived her husband.
> Her prayers were not answered immediately.

Sarah
>She had to wait an un-thinkable amount of time for her blessing (I thought 10 years was a long time – not compared to 90!)
>She had trouble believing God's promises to her.
>She doubted what God could do through her.
>She attempted to work problems out on her own, without consulting God.
>She tried to cover her own faults by blaming others.
>She lied to God.

Elizabeth
>She experienced loneliness and public shame.
>She had to wait for God's timing instead of her own.

Rachel
>Her envy and competitiveness marred her relationship with her sister.
>She was dishonest.
>She failed to recognize that her husband's devotion was not dependent on her ability to have children.
>She was jealous and unforgiving.

After reading about these women, I found myself feeling relieved that I wasn't the only one God "picked on." I find it interesting that just the same is true for a lady named Elizabeth who wrote the following:

"I faced the future of an empty womb while those women of the Bible, who were supposed to encourage me, became fruitful. Sarah, Hannah, Elizabeth and the rest of their sorority had received a 'yes' to their prayer requests. Yet, the results of my prayers were as negative as all of the pregnancy tests I had ever taken.

What I needed to see was God giving someone a 'No' answer. It was then God laid 2 Corinthians 12:7-9 on my heart. I, too, had a thorn in the flesh, a physical condition that pricked my heart. I, too, had prayed to have it removed and was told 'No'. I took comfort in God's answer to Paul, 'My grace is sufficient for you, for my power is made perfect in weakness.'

I began to follow Paul's example, appreciating the work God could do in me because of the weakness of infertility… not just in spite of it." [3]

Another woman named Ruth withstood three years of hearing "no" from God. Then He revealed a verse tucked away in the Old Testament that helped her climb out of the "pit" of secondary infertility: *"One day I took out my Bible to search for some words of comfort. I was going to look in the Book of John, but my Bible opened to the Book of Zephaniah instead. My eyes were drawn to a verse that had been underlined on the page. It was my Bible, so I had to have underlined this verse, but I have no idea why, when or where. It was verse 3:17—'The Lord your God is with you, he is mighty to save. He will take great delight in you, he will quiet you with his love, he will rejoice over you with singing.' I wrote in the margin of my Bible that day, 'what a reassurance.' I feel like I've gotten a letter from God and I want to read it over and over again."*

God is the great mercy giver, isn't He!

"Arming" Yourself with the Word

Why is it so important to read your Bible daily? There are several answers and the number one answer is: God commands you to.

A great example of how the Bible will benefit you lies in Ephesians 6:10-20. It explains how to "wear the whole armor of God." Paul tells us in verse 11 to *"Put on all of God's armor so that you will be able to stand safe against all strategies and tricks of Satan. For we are not fighting against people made of flesh and blood, but against persons without bodies – the evil rulers of the unseen world..." (NLT)*

Before I explain the "armor," I want you to realize that if you are a new believer or you are new to the Bible, you are considered a "baby Christian." When you were a baby, your mother fed you milk, not meat and potatoes. The same is true of baby Christians; they start out learning the basics (1 Peter 2:2-3) and then move on to the "meat" which includes the "armor" of God as well as spiritual warfare, which is explained in the next chapter. If you have difficulty interpreting this information, I suggest you consult the clergy of your church.

I want you to understand why God speaks often about the devil in the Bible. It's because He wants you to be prepared for your "spiritual fight." In His infinite wisdom, He used the analogy of a soldier's uniform to describe how you can defend yourself against Satan. To put it in simple terms, the Armor of God is using the Bible as the ultimate defense. Reading it *daily* gives you:

Understanding of the truth—Belt of truth
Obedience to the truth—Breastplate of righteousness
Assurance in the truth of your salvation—Helmet of Salvation

Faith in the truth (especially during trials)—Shield of Faith
The ability to share the truth (witnessing)—Gospel of Peace
Truth as a weapon to fight back with—Sword of the Spirit

Because the evil one does exist and he does try to defeat you through lies, through setbacks, during periods of vulnerability, and through his schemes, you are wise to "arm" yourself with knowledge of the truth – it is your weapon. Let's put it this way: Once you understand God's Word, you can interpret truth from lies. When Lucifer attacks your heart (your self worth and emotions) God's approval, which is the breastplate protects this vital organ.

When it seems too risky or scary to tell others about Jesus, His "shoes" give you the motivation to share the free gift of salvation. The Bible acts like a shield that enables your faith to grow. When the devil makes you doubt God or your salvation, put on the helmet to *protect your mind*. Satan sees you as a threat and you use the truth to defeat him—by using your sword. If you don't read the Bible, you miss step one and you're unable to put on the rest of the armor. You'll be defeated sooner or later.

This is a very deep subject and one I advise you to learn about, especially during the trials in your life. Once again, I advise you to seek further instruction from your pastor or priest, a Bible study group, spiritual leaders, or go to the "man upstairs" and pray for wisdom.

Speaking of praying, the seventh aspect of the "armor of God" is prayer. Ephesians 6:18 reads *"Pray all the time. Ask God for anything in line with Holy Spirit's wishes. Plead with him, reminding him of your needs, and keep praying earnestly for all Christians everywhere."* (NLT)

The best advice I can offer is that you to write to receive monthly or quarterly devotions named *Our Daily Bread*. They are very short daily readings that have corresponding verses for you to look up and learn from. To receive these devotions, go to **www.odb.org or write to: RBC Ministries, PO Box 2222, Grand Rapids, MI 49501-2222**. Make a pattern of reading your devotion and then praying daily.

Learning How to Pray

Prayer is very powerful as you can see by Rebekah's story. If you're like me, you walk into an empty room and automatically turn on the television or radio for background noise to drown out the quiet. Try leaving them off and asking God to converse with you. As you race across town or down the highway, turn off the radio and tell him you want to talk. Believe it or not, this is prayer. Don't be

CHAPTER 4—READING THE BIBLE AND PRAYING DAILY

distracted by billboards and fast food signs. Pull your attention back and say something like *I'm sorry God, I got distracted. I'm back now. What do you want to share with me?*

Talk to God about how you woke up with a headache, or your husband was less than cordial. Or better yet, how the smell of bacon, or dew on the grass smells so wonderful. Go to the all-the-time listener instead of your mother, your girlfriends, or your cohorts at work. You could fall into a trap of gossip, disenchantment, or negativism that way.

If I were to stop typing right now and call my friend on the phone, I would probably say something like, *what's up? How was your day? What did you do?* We would share feelings, concerns and accomplishments with each other. In my opinion, praying is the same. It's what God wants most from us – our thoughts, dreams, disappointments, concerns and most of all, our thanks.

It is perfectly fine to ask the Lord for a baby or even more babies. Just remind yourself that His answer may be "yes," it may be "no," or perhaps it will be "yes, but later." What's important is asking and not demanding; asking with good motives; asking and then accepting. What if He blesses you with a child requiring special needs? Are you prepared for that? What if you adopt a child and you don't bond immediately? Are you willing to make the effort to learn to fall in love with him or her? Be prepared to accept the answers to what you pray for.

I want to also point out that while growing up, I recited prayers that had been written for me. I'm grateful that I was praying and that I knew whom God the Father, Jesus His Son, and the Holy Spirit were, nevertheless, God tells us in Matthew 6:7, that He dislikes recited prayer.

Instead, He wants us to talk to Him in an open, honest manner. Sometimes I find myself praying to God from the point of a daughter seeking confirmation and direction from Her Heavenly Father. Other times I tell Him my complaints, fears and frustrations. Some of my prayers offer Him thanks and praise and some include hopes, wishes and desires. Even though He resides within you and knows what you are thinking, He wants you to demonstrate faith and reverence by praying to Him.

Because He knew we wouldn't know how to approach Him, God so compassionately and lovingly gave us the Lord's Prayer[4] (you'll find it in Matthew 6:9-13), as *an example* of how to pray. He didn't intend for us to recite it word for word, instead, He wants one-on-one chats with us.

You may be thinking, I have been praying and nothing is happening. I understand. Unanswered prayer made me feel like the lover of my soul was uninterested; I began to wonder if He had forgotten me. On the contrary, unanswered prayer doesn't necessarily mean "no;" it might mean, wait.

God is quite aware that we humans hate waiting. We are accustomed to instant gratification. The Lord is wise and He knows that waiting makes us cling to Him. It forces us to persevere. God may decide to withhold his answer for a while – this does not mean He is ignoring you. His delay may be intended to: 1) deepen your insight into what you really need, 2) broaden your appreciation for his answers, or 3) allow you to mature so you can use his answers wisely.

Let me point out another mistake I made and you should avoid. I stumbled upon the following verse and tried to distort it to my benefit: *"Until now you have not asked for anything in my name. Ask and you will receive, and your joy will be complete."* (John 16:24.)

I read that verse and I thought I had it made. All I had to do was pray for a child *in Christ's name* and I would receive. Poof, I expected to be pregnant the next month. After all, I truly believed in God and I asked in all faith and sincerity.

The baby didn't come and I was confused. Was this verse a lie? No, it wasn't. In hindsight, I know that God did answer my prayers. I asked to give birth to a child. God wanted my husband and I to adopt. I wanted the child NOW!!! The children He had selected for us hadn't been conceived yet. I asked in Jesus' name and I received, just not in the manner nor the time table I had envisioned. I had to learn that His plan is always perfect and complete!

John and Earl share their own experiences with prayer: *"My wife and I know that our infertility struggle has helped us to grow in our prayer life, for we have come to realize how utterly dependent we are on God. It has helped us in our trust, for we know that the God who has helped us resolve our infertility struggle, will see us through the rest of life as well. It has helped us grow in our sensitivity to the suffering of others, for our infertility has placed us in contact with many others who have an infertility problem, but who have not yet reached their point of resolution."* John[5]

Earl asked, *"Why did our son have to die? If God loves us, why does He let tragedies happen? Had I angered God? Upon reflection,"* he said, *"I realized that I sinned against Him continually. On the other hand, I knew God was good, and despite how I felt and hurt, I believed He would bring good out this bad situation.*

The answers to my questions came... as I turned to the Bible for inspiration. At first, no passage seemed appropriate. Then I remembered a verse I had memorized years ago, but its impact was different this time. In the Gospel of

John, Jesus Christ spoke to a bewildered Nicodemus about how a person must be born again of the Spirit to be saved. He explained the divine plan: 'For God so loved the world that He gave his one and only Son. Whomever believes in Him shall not perish but have eternal life,' (John 3:16). As my attention was drawn to the first part of the verse, it was as if the Spirit of God had put His hand on my shoulder, saying to my heart, 'I know what it is like to lose a son.'

God did not explain why our son had to die. He didn't give me answers; He gave me Himself. He alone is sufficient for our needs and our wounds. At a time when I was spiritually broken, He dealt with me graciously, according to His own principles described in the Bible.

As I prayed earnestly with a 'mustard seed' of faith, broken in spirit, utterly dependent on Him, and confessing my sinfulness, God used His Word to counsel and comfort me, and to teach me about Himself. When I came to Him on His terms—not mine—His Word came alive.

I had lost my son involuntarily and would have preferred to have it otherwise. God gave His Son voluntarily for you and me, and He would not have had it any other way." [6]

When you finally have your answers you can usually look back at the trial and realize like Paul did, *"...that what has happened to me has really served to advance the gospel,"* (Philippians 1:12).

"The Lord is good to those whose hope is in him, to the one who seeks him..." Lamentations 3:25

Pray Without Ceasing

Now that you know how to pray, practice daily. Make praying a habit in your life. You probably eat breakfast every day, or perhaps you start the day with a cup of coffee, hot chocolate or tea. Just add praying to that pattern and I guarantee you'll notice a difference in your life. Here are six additional pieces of advice concerning prayer:

1. In your prayers, *worship the Father*. Notice the first two lines of "The Lord's Prayer" give honor at the beginning of them: *"Our Father in heaven, Hallowed be your name."* "Hallowed" basically means you honor His holy name.

2. *Ask for God's will to be done.* It's easy to inform God of what you don't have or what you want. You may even find yourself trying to change *His* mind. Remember, He knows the big picture, and He promises many times that He wants to bless you abundantly. Remember though, abundant may mean a life of plenty or it may mean a life of challenges that motivate you to consider options you hadn't considered or planned for.

3. John 14:13 tells us, *"And I will do whatever you ask in my name, so that the Son may bring glory to the Father."* Consider beginning your prayers with something like, "Dear Jesus," or ending them with "in Jesus' name." These are just examples; you will know what feels natural to you. Remember, if you pray in Jesus' name for something that is not His will don't be disappointed. The two go hand in hand, and His plan will be revealed to you in time.

4. In 1 Thessalonians 5:17 we are commanded to *pray without ceasing.* Be persistent in your prayers. Persistence demonstrates faith that God will answer. Faith shouldn't die if the answers don't come immediately; for the delay may be God's way of working his will in your life.

Furthermore, I always thought that I had to be alone and kneeling for God to hear my prayers. Reverence is wonderful. Solitude, submission and meditation are excellent ingredients for prayer. But we don't always have that luxury. So, pray where you are: in the car, on the telephone with a friend, in bed. Just pray!

5. Give thanks. Tell God all what you are thankful for. If you can't think of anything, thank Him for your life, your husband, your food, water, air, and so on. When you really get to know Him, you'll even be able to thank Him for this trial because you will understand that it has made your relationship with Him more personal, your faith stronger, and your understanding of His perfect plan for your life more intense.

6. When you are mature in your Christian walk, learn to *pray specifically* like Eliezer did in Rebekah's story (Genesis 24:14 NLT). Notice how he gave God the opportunity to answer his prayer: *"This is my request: When I ask one of them for a drink and she says, 'Yes, certainly, and I will water your camels too!'—let her be the one you have appointed as Isaac's wife. That is how I will know."*

A modern-day example of praying specifically could be something like… *Lord, if it is your will that I have Artificial Insemination, I pray in Jesus' name, that in the next week my husband will bring up the subject and ask me*

CHAPTER 4—READING THE BIBLE AND PRAYING DAILY

to consider it. Remember, you are asking for God's plan, so do not try to change His mind, or make Him aware, or test Him. If you don't get the answer you want, don't be upset, be thankful that your prayers were answered.

Claudia prayed to the Lord and was amazed at his response: *"Four and a half years ago, the idea of adopting had never even crossed my mind. My husband, Bob, and I had four wonderful kids so I believed my family was complete. However, three little words and God's gentle nudge changed everything.*

I had just met a mom from our church named Jan who, at that time, had adopted four children from Russia. I thought that was very special and told her what a really worthwhile thing she was doing. She answered back with three little words: 'You could adopt.' Of course, I had MANY reasons why adopting was impossible for us. Living on just Bob's salary as a teacher in a small home with four children already topped the list. Yet the thought just wouldn't go away. I fought it. I began to pray about it – constantly – trying to argue with God why the idea was crazy.

I never spoke a single word to Bob about my thoughts or struggles with God. At one point, Jan mentioned she and her husband were praying for us to consider adopting. She suggested I just talk to my husband about it. I told her if God wanted us to adopt, HE could talk to Bob. I know this sounds flippant, but that was how I felt. I wasn't about to have this be another of my harebrained ideas. Still, God's nudging continued. Finally, I gave up. Second Chronicles 1:7b says, '...ask for whatever you want me to give to you.' Citing that verse, I asked God to please give me more children if it was his will and I thanked him for the precious blessings already entrusted to our care.

Afterward coincidences continued to pile up – all having to do with Russia and adopting (I documented in my journal 27 in all!) It got to the point where I finally confided my confusion about what God was doing to a close friend. I told her that if Bob ever got the idea to adopt on his own, I would know it was from God. THAT VERY NIGHT as we were discussing the Russian dancers who were set to perform at church, Bob mentioned that if it were up to him, he'd adopt in a minute. My mouth surely dropped open, and later I rushed to our garage for privacy to phone my friend and ask her to pray for us. At that point, I KNEW that we would eventually adopt.

Now we have four more kids in our family to love: Vova and Marina from St. Petersburg, Russia, and Val and Sveta who came home from the Ukraine this past March. Though we've had our share of difficulties in trying to become a family, I KNOW beyond a shadow of a doubt that God brought us together and He will use this for His glory. I've felt enormous peace knowing we're abiding in God's will. In one translation of Jeremiah 29:11, God says, 'I know what I am planning for you... I have good plans for you, not plans to hurt you. I will give you a hope and a good future.' Jesus also says in Luke 9:48, 'Whoever welcomes this little child in my name, welcomes me...'

We still live only on Bob's salary, and now we have eight kids between the ages of 11 and 16 living in our 1800 sq. ft. house. Yet we are blessed beyond measure. Second Corinthians 9:8 reads, 'And God is able to make all grace abound to you, so that in all things at all times, having all that you need, you will abound in every good work.' That's a lot of ALLs, and I've seen firsthand that this is true. I am so very thankful for the work God is doing in all of us and that He gave us the opportunity to completely change for kids' lives, both now and for all eternity."

When you make a habit of praying daily, you will enjoy it. Evidentially it takes 21 days to establish a habit. Try in earnest to pray daily for three weeks and you'll get to the point where it is a part of your life.

How Your Prayers are Hindered

"There is no power like that of prevailing, spirit energized and directed prayer. It changes things. It changes circumstances, situations and events. It changes people, both those being prayed for and those doing the praying, turning ordinary mortals into people of power. It brings power. It brings wisdom. It brings life. It brings peace. It brings God!" said Faye Powell, one of the founders of the church I attend.

When teaching about prayer at a women's retreat in April of 1997, Mrs. Powell continued: *"When we, as far as we know, have been living in obedience to the Word of God, there is joy in our prayer life. We like to spend time with our Father, and we see results in answers to our prayers. But when disobedience and unbelief creep in, the joy goes out of those treasured times together, such as when a child avoids eye contact with a parent to whom he's been disobedient, and the fellowship is broken. These things hinder your prayers:*

Unconfessed sin both known and unknown—*"If I had cherished sin in my heart, the Lord would not have listened; but God has surely listened and*

CHAPTER 4—READING THE BIBLE AND PRAYING DAILY

heard my voice in prayer," Psalm 66:18.

Unbelief—*"And without faith it is impossible to please God, because anyone who comes to him must believe that he exists and that he rewards those who earnestly seek him,"* Hebrews 11:6

Unforgiveness—*"For if you forgive men when they sin against you, your Heavenly Father will also forgive you. But if you do not forgive men their sins, your Father will not forgive your sins,"* Matthew 6:14-15

Disobedience—*"If you remain in me and my words remain in you, ask whatever you wish, and it will be given you,"* John 15:7.

Unstable mind—*"But when he asks, he must believe and not doubt, because he who doubts is like a wave of the sea, blown and tossed by the wind,"* James 1:6-7.

Self-seeking motive—*"When you ask you do not receive, because you ask with wrong motives, that you may spend what you get on your pleasures,"* James 4:3.

She concluded, *"Sometimes we come to prayer doubting that we dare to turn loose of our desires and ask God to do it HIS way. What if He leads us contrary to our deepest desires? Is that okay? Can we trust His wisdom? Can we really trust His father-love for us?"* Only you can answer that.

To say your prayers are hindered means sin is causing a separation between you and God. Because the sin is unconfessed, He cannot hear your prayers, protect you, or bless you. It is always important and wise to take a "spiritual evaluation" of yourself and determine if you are "clean" before the Lord. Remember, He delights in you and He longs to bless you richly.

***"But your iniquities have separated you from your God; your sins have hidden his face from you, so that he will not hear."* Isaiah 59:2**

Chapter Five—Identifying Unconfessed Sin

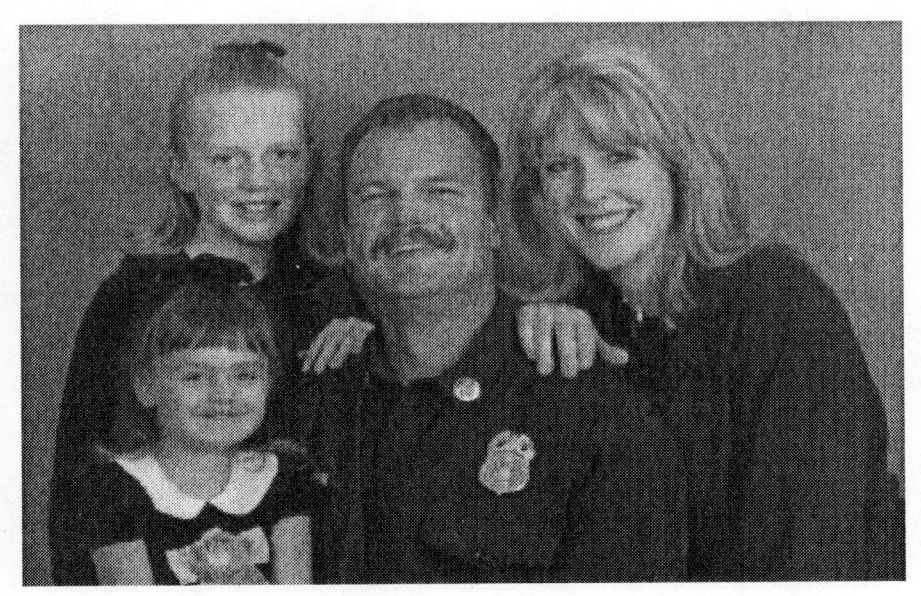

Christine and Sarah with Brian and Susan

-Meeting the "Lion"
    Addressing the Lies
    Fear is the Root of Most Sin
    Unconfessed Sin and Unanswered Prayer
-Exposing the Idols of Obsession, Pride and Pity
    Obsession— A Silent Idol
    Pride—Let the Walls Fall Down
    Poor, Poor Pitiful Me
    How to Fight Back

Chapter Five–Identifying Unconfessed Sin

1. When your period comes and you are upset and disappointed, how do you handle it? (Take a bubble bath and calm down? Call your husband and cry? Seclude yourself at home? Go out in public and pretend nothing is wrong? Get on your knees and pray?)

_____

_____

_____

2. Do you struggle with pride when it comes to infertility? Yes or No? If so, in what areas? (Faking happiness? Not relying on God? Building "walls" of protection? Being rude to others?)

_____

_____

_____

3. Do you know what a pity party is? Yes or No? If so, please describe it:

_____

_____

_____

4. Is there sin in your life that you refuse to confess? Yes or No? If yes, please list it:

_____

_____

_____

Stop and seriously consider confessing it NOW.

5. Is there someone in your life whom you refuse to forgive? Yes or No? If yes, please list all of them:

_____

_____

_____

Stop and consider calling them right NOW.

6. Do you believe Satan exists? Yes or No? Do you believe hell exists? Yes or No?

7. Do you realize that God doesn't tempt you to sin, but Satan does? Yes or No? Do you realize that you are most vulnerable to temptation when you are discouraged? Yes or No?

8. Do you ever wonder if God is punishing you? Yes or No? If yes, why would He do that?

_____

_____

_____

9. Do you feel God has deserted you in your "hour of need?" Yes or No?

10. Do you find yourself playing "mind games?" If so, what do they sound like? Please describe:

_____

_____

_____

11. Has infertility ever gotten you depressed enough to consider suicide? Yes or No?

Recommended Reading:

Psalm 66:10
John 8:42-27, 10:10
2 Corinthians 2:9-11
Philippians 4:8
2 Thessalonians 1:9-10
Hebrews 12:1-4
2 Peter 2:19b
Revelation 12:7-10, 20:10

Isaiah 14:12-17
1 Corinthians 10:13
Ephesians 6:10-20
Colossians 1:13
2 Timothy 2:12
1 Peter 5:8
1 John 1:8-10, 4:4

Look up these verses and fill in the blanks:

2 Thessalonians 1:9 (NLT): *"They will be punished in everlasting hell, forever _____ from the Lord, never to see the glory of his power."*

Revelation 12:9 (NLT): *"This great dragon – the ancient serpent called the devil, or _____, the one deceiving the whole world – was thrown down onto the earth with all his _____."*

James 4:7 (NLT): *"So give yourselves humbly to God. Resist the devil and he will _____ from you."*

"Why Aren't You Listening to Me God?"
Answer #4—A barren womb helps you identify unconfessed sin in your life that results in unanswered prayer and separation from the guidance and protection of your heavenly Father.

Chapter 5—Sarah's Story

I always wanted to be a mother. I just expected to conceive after my marriage to Abraham. When it didn't happen at first I was confused. During my day women got married and had babies. We didn't have college educations, careers or support groups for the barren.

It seemed like a lifetime of waiting for our family to grow. Finally when Abe was 99 years old, the Lord told him he would bless us with a son to inherit our estate. In fact, he said Abraham's descendants would be like the stars in the sky – "too many to count." It was so hard for us to fathom. I had faith in God, but Abe's faith was much stronger than mine.

After I heard the news, I knew I was too old to bear a child, so I surmised God had something else in mind. I thought God would send a son through another woman – a common practice in Israel. So, I decided to have my husband sleep with my slave girl, Hagar, and I would raise the child as my own. It seemed like no big deal. I wasn't hurting anyone. After all, God said he was sending us a son.

I couldn't have been more wrong. After Hagar became pregnant, she turned on me! I was so angry I beat her. It was all Abe's fault. He should have never slept with her!

Sarah gave Hagar to Abraham as a substitute wife, a perfectly acceptable practice at that time. A married woman who could not have children was shamed by her peers and was often required to give a female servant to her husband in order to produce heirs. The children born to the servant woman were considered the children of the wife. Abraham was acting in line with the custom of the day. But his action showed a lack of faith in God to fulfill his promise that Abraham and Sarah would have a child.

By taking matters into her own hands and "helping God," Sarah experienced many problems. She blamed her husband for her own actions; she later lied; her servant girl treated her poorly; and, she ended up mistreating Hagar.

Because Sarah did have faith, she gave birth to a baby boy when she was 90 years old and Abraham was 100.[1]

"Sarah, too, had faith, and because of this she was able to become a mother in spite of her old age, for she realized that God, who gave her his promise would certainly do what he said." **Hebrews 11:11 (NLT)**

Meeting the "Lion"

I fell head first into the enemy's snare. Yes, God's enemy, Satan, is the ruler of this world *for now* and his intentions are clear: to steal, kill and destroy. He's after each one of us because his time is short. He intends to steal your joy, kill your marriage, and destroy your relationship with Christ. If you haven't given your heart to Jesus, he wants to make sure you never do. Beware my friends. Read Revelation 12:9 for more about the Father of Lies.

This book is intended to intensify your relationship with Jesus Christ, so I do not want to give Satan an inch of glory. However it is very important that you are aware of his schemes, lies and tempting. In Matthew 12:30, Jesus says, *"He who is not with me is against me; and he who does not gather with me scatters."* Ladies, there is no third choice. It's either love God or love Satan. Once you are more aware of his role in this world you will be better prepared for his attacks. (2 Corinthians 2:11.)[2]

The "snare" I referred to occurs when we take our eyes off Jesus and place them on ourselves, our needs, and what we DON'T have—essentially ignoring the blessings God provides. Look at the example in 2 Corinthians 11:3—*"But I am afraid that just as Eve was deceived by the serpent's cunning, your minds may somehow be led astray from your sincere and pure devotion to Christ."* Vulnerability is at the root of the issue. First Peter 5:8 warns us that the enemy is a roaring lion waiting to devour anyone who is vulnerable. You see, I was vulnerable; wake up my friend—so are you!

After I was snared I stepped right into the enemy's "foothold" (*a secure position*).[3] Let me explain this. The snare was listening too long when the enemy constantly reminded me of what I was missing. I stopped looking up and repeatedly looked in the mirror for guidance and support. Another way to look at footholds, in my opinion, is by considering them like an invitation. For example, my resentment toward my husband grew to the point that I basically *invited* Satan to take a secure position in my life. Of course, I didn't recognize this until after the fact.

The foothold gave way to a stronghold *(a fortress,)*[4] when I became obsessed with becoming a mother. There wasn't a minute in the day when I wasn't feeling sorry for myself. The aching I felt for a child was so strong I stopped going out. By secluding myself at home, I fell into depression and pity—ripe territory for the enemy.

Bondage (*the condition of a slave*)[5] took over when pride reared its ugly head. I hadn't completely given my life to Christ yet, so the Holy Spirit didn't reside in me to advise me of good choices. I wasn't covered by God's "umbrella" of protection. Sin was the root of the problem and I didn't even realize it. Even though I was seeking God through church attendance, Bible study and even prayer, my eyes were on myself. When I finally placed the Lord on the "throne" of my life and let Him take control, my prayers were heard once again, the blood Jesus sacrificed cleansed me of my sins, and the Prince of Darkness was defeated.

I am referring to "spiritual warfare" here —a term that was foreign to me, and one that seemed a little spooky. Looking back, I can picture God and His enemy fighting over me (just like He fights for you). Satan and his demons (1/3 of the angels who left heaven with him—see Isaiah 14:12-15,)[6] rule this world until Christ's return.

In the meantime, they seek out the vulnerable and they attack them in their greatest areas of vulnerability. The attacks take the form of physical ailments, depression, difficult times, anger, jealousy, temptations, and more. He knows our "hot buttons" and he pushes them to trip us up and make us sin. He can't be everywhere at once and he's definitely not all knowing, but he can certainly wreak havoc in this world.

On the other hand, God and His angels have already won the victory over you. When Jesus died on the cross, Satan was defeated. Until Christ returns, the devil battles with God for your soul. Even though you can't see it, He and His angels battle with Lucifer and his demons constantly over you (Ephesians 6:12.)[7]

Have you had these thoughts whispered in your ear before: *Why me? Where are you God? If you love me so much Lord, how could you allow me to hurt like this? Am I being punished? Does God think I'm not worthy to be a mother? Maybe I should just divorce my husband so he can marry someone who can give him children. I should just make it easier on everyone and end my life.*

The great deceiver sees an opportunity to cause turmoil in your life, so he fills you with these thoughts and lies. When you aren't prepared, he subtly

CHAPTER 5—IDENTIFYING UNCONFESSED SIN

and seductively creates confusion in your life because he wants you to curse God. The reason for this chapter is to teach you how to be prepared.

These are the ways the enemy tries to trick you:

* Self focus	* Shame	* Discontent
* Temptation	* Unforgiveness	* Suicidal thoughts
* Self pity	* Resentment	* Pride
* Anger	* Jealousy	* Restlessness

Does any of this sound familiar? It's scary, but now that you know he's tempting you with sin you can fight back. Here's how:

When you are fed lies, **remind him that he has already lost the battle**. Tell him Galatians 2:20a—*"I have been crucified with Christ..."*

Guard your thoughts and your mind. To do this, stay away from negativism, evil or impurity. Put good things into your mind. Be aware of your surroundings. Choose television programs and movies carefully. Something that has really helped me, is switching from a secular radio station to a Christian station. The one I chose can be heard around the world – it is Air 1 and you can check out their website at www.Air1.com.

Take your thoughts captive. When a thought comes into your mind that is ugly or untrue, instead of entertaining it, purposely kick it out by thinking of something else. Remind yourself of something pleasant such as your favorite verse or how much you are loved.

Place your eyes on Christ by reading His Word and praying daily. Ask the Lord to talk to you through His Holy Spirit during your prayer and reading times.

Don't give the enemy your attention. Think on what is pleasant, pure and lovely.

Resist temptation by choosing obedience.

If you feel like you are in bondage or that the enemy is after you, take courage and strength in the Lord. Don't give up. Your faith will be tested, but you have God's Word to use as your weapon. Infertility is the vice grip the enemy has on you now, but you can turn it around by faith and give glory to God.

Whatever the outcome, whether it is advanced testing or procedures, putting off testing to work on your marriage, foster care, adoption, or continuing your marriage as a complete family, it is imperative that you hand this burden over to God and leave it with Him. Don't take it back. Leave it there and allow yourself to heal. The goal from here on out should be to get to a point where you will gladly and freely accept the plan God has for you, even if it is nurturing children instead of raising them.

Addressing the Lies

I want to go back and address the thoughts and lies the enemy often whispers to women experiencing fertility issues. The first one in the previous list was:

Why me? My answer is, why not you? Everyone experiences adversities in their lives. Look around. People are dealing with devastating diseases such as AIDS and cancer; spouses are learning of infidelity in their marriages; others are dealing with the loss of a loved one. This *is your* trial.

Where are you God? In 2 Corinthians 1:3, 4 (NLT) Paul says, *"...What a wonderful God we have – he is the Father of our Lord Jesus Christ, the source of every mercy, and the one who so wonderfully comforts and strengthens us in our hardships and trials. And why does he do this? So that when others are troubled, needing our sympathy and encouragement, we can pass on to them this same help and comfort God has given us."*

Now notice the second part of this verse: *"And why does he do this? So that when others are troubled, needing our sympathy and encouragement, we can pass on to them this same help and comfort God has given us."* Other people in your life will experience trials of their own and once you've learned about faith and trust, you will be able to extend a helping hand to them.

If you love me so much Lord, how can you allow me to hurt like this? In Psalm 138:7a (NLT), David said to the Lord: *"Though I am surrounded by troubles, you will bring me safely through them."* Hold fast to this verse. Remember, God's Word is full of promises. So far, none of them have been broken and I believe they never will be. For some it takes a "step of faith" to accept Jesus into their life, for others it takes a "leap." Now, it will take faith to believe God knows what he's doing regarding your maternal instincts.

Am I being punished? Many women (and couples) find themselves wondering if God is punishing them for promiscuity earlier in their lives, affairs, or abortions. I believe there are consequences to sin that we can't avoid, but if we confess and repent, we are forgiven and our sins are erased. If they are erased, then how can God keep punishing us for them? Often He forgives us, but we don't forgive ourselves.

On the other hand, if you have unconfessed sin in your life, then you are not right with God and your prayers are not heard (1 Peter 3:7; Matthew 5:23, 24; 1 John 4:20). It is imperative that you confess any past sins with a contrite heart. Remind yourself that no sin is too big to be forgiven. Once you take care of your past with God, the lines of communication between you and Him will be opened up once again. At this point, do not allow Satan to pester you with regretful memories.

Does God think I'm not worthy to be a mother? This is a tough question that I wrestled with often. When you see a child killed by their parents on the evening news or you witness someone abusing their child in a public restroom, it's only natural to wonder about the fairness of life. The answer remains the same – only God knows the plans He has for *you*. I believe that when He places a desire for children in your heart, He fulfills that desire one way or another. We will address some of those ways in Chapter 10. For now, only time will tell.

Maybe I should just divorce my husband so he can marry someone who can give him children. This thought came to me so many times. I'm so glad I didn't fall for this lie. The enemy would love one less Christian marriage in this world and one less opportunity for children to grow up in a Christian home. Don't even entertain this lure. Talk to your husband so he will be aware of the pressure you are feeling. He may be able to help comfort and reassure you, if not, consider seeing a counselor and above all, ask the Lord to restrain Satan from you.

I should just make it easier on everyone and end my life. This thought also came to me quite often. After our first adoption fell through, I sat on my bed, at home, for hours pondering the thought that a loaded gun lay inches away from me in a safe that I knew the combination to. The sheer frustration of it all was too much to bear. Then I replaced that thought and considered Job. To describe what happened to him, I want you to read his story starting at Job 1:1—

"In the land of Uz there lived a man whose name was Job. This man was blameless and upright; he feared God and shunned evil. He had seven sons and three daughters, and he owned 7,000 sheep, 3,000 camels, 500 yoke of oxen and 500 donkeys and had a large number of servants. He was the greatest man among all the people of the East."

Job 1:9-11—*One day Satan went to God and said, "Does Job fear God for nothing? Have you not put a hedge around him and his household and everything he has? You have blessed the work of his hands, so that his flocks and herds are spread throughout the land. But stretch out your hand and strike everything he has, and he will surely curse you to your face."*

Job 1:12—*"The Lord said to Satan, 'Very well, then, everything he has is in your hands, but on the man himself do not lay a finger."* Job 1:21—Satan destroyed everything Job had including his family. When Job found out, he said, *"Naked I came from my mother's womb, and naked I will depart. The Lord gave and the Lord has taken away; may the name of the Lord be praised."*

Is Satan evil, or what? He set this man up to curse God and luckily, he failed. He would love nothing more than to set you up too and eventually convince you to commit suicide. If you were a Christian, there would be one less believer in the world; if you were not, there would be one more person on his side; your husband and family would be left devastated which he could use for *his* glory; and if you had children, there would be one less complete family to contend with.

Notice how Satan accused God of forming a "hedge" around Job. As I understand, this means a boundary or circle of angels protecting Job and his "household." You can pray for a "hedge of protection" around you, your marriage and your household. Take every measure to make sure Satan's evil plans for you do not come to fruition.

Fear is the Root of Most Sin

"I said, 'You are my servant'; I have chosen you and have not rejected you. So do not fear, for I am with you; do not be dismayed, for I am your God. I will strengthen you and help you; I will uphold you with my righteous right hand." **Isaiah 41:9c-10**

When it comes to this trial, what is it that you fear most? Is it time getting away from you? Is it feeling "different" the rest of your life? Is it realizing that you will never feel life within you? Are you afraid to adopt "someone else's child?" Are you afraid God isn't blessing you with a second child because He's not pleased with the job you have done with the first? Are you afraid your marriage isn't strong enough to carry on as a family of two? When you are feeling anxious about an issue, you are holding the problem in your hand and not allowing God access to it.

You are not alone. Many people in the Bible experienced fear just like you do. According to *The Living Bible*,[8] God said *"don't be afraid"* to each one of these godly people as they experienced fear:

Abraham—Genesis 15:1
Moses—Numbers 21:34 and Deuteronomy 3:2
Joshua—Joshua 8:1
Jeremiah—Lamentations 3:57
Daniel—Daniel 10:12, 19
Zacharias—Luke 1:13
Mary—Luke 1:30
Shepherds—Luke 2:10
Peter—Luke 5:10
Paul—Acts 27:24
John—Revelation 1:17, 18

Everyone experiences fear. My fear was of the unknown. I was afraid my husband would leave me... afraid that I might be a terrible mother... afraid I would be the only one in town with this terrible "disease." Of the many fears, I was afraid most of becoming a bitter, old lady. No one likes to be around such a person; they are angry people and they are not a lot of fun. Perhaps that is why I inadvertently chose the opposite extreme—faking happiness.

When you choose to ignore underlying fear, the enemy uses **disappointment, discouragement, depression, dejection and demoralization** to spiral you downward. *He does this in your mind.* Janet recounts the "mind games" she played with herself while experiencing secondary infertility:

"One mind game I played was this: Whenever I found out somebody was pregnant, I would think to myself, well, there goes my chance this month. God gave that baby to them."

Janet admits the worst mind game she played concerned her faith. She grew up in a very dedicated Catholic household where her family went to church every Sunday. "*Life was good to me,*" she recalled. Janet recounts leading a perfect life – until she became a Christian. Suddenly she had trouble getting pregnant and when she did conceive, miscarriage followed.

Guilt made her wonder if God was punishing her for leaving the Catholic Church—the church her parents raised her in. *"I wondered if I was being a bad girl and committing a sin for going against my parents' beliefs,"* she confessed.

Do you see how Satan craftfully twisted circumstances to make Janet second guess herself? He is very sneaky and he loves to cause chaos in our lives. When your mind is jumbled with confusion, you lack the clarity that God desires for you. So, go back to question number 10 and look at the list of mind games you listed. Take a dark pencil or marker and cross them out. Never allow them to return and be mindful to kick them out of your brain if they try to re-enter.

When Satan wages war in your mind, read 2 Corinthians 10:3-5 [9] – the way to fight back is to take your thoughts *captive*. When a thought such as *You can't be trusted with a baby,* comes into your mind, instead of entertaining it, tell your mind to kick it out. And then tell yourself all of the things you learned about God's love for you in Chapter 4.

Let's address another area of fear – it's called worrying. I've wasted so much time worrying about money, the unknown, health, and the future throughout my life. I'll never forget the day when my husband was in veterinary school and I was fretting over bills. He looked at me and said, *"Why do you worry so much? Don't you really believe God is taking care of you and providing for all of your needs? Where is your faith?"*

Of course, I thought he was attacking my character at the time and my response was very defensive, however, once that thought was planted in my mind, the Holy Spirit began revealing how my lack of faith was offensive to God. *The Living Bible* lists seven reasons not to worry;[10] they are taken from verses in the Book of Matthew:

- The same God who created life in you can be trusted with the details of your life, (vs. 6:26).
- Worrying about the future hampers your efforts for today, (vs. 6:26).
- Worrying is more harmful than helpful, (vs. 6:27).
- God does not ignore those who depend on Him, (vs. 6:28-30).
- Worry shows a lack of faith and understanding of God, (vs. 6:32).
- There are real challenges God wants us to pursue, and worrying keeps us from them, (vs. 6:33).
- Living one day at a time keeps us from being consumed with worry, (vs. 6:34).

Because of its ill effects, Jesus tells us in verse 6:25 not to worry about those needs that God promises to supply. Worry causes the following effects:[11]

- It affects you physically—making you unable to sleep or eat (remember Hannah?).
- It causes the object of your worry to consume your thoughts (remember my testimony?).

CHAPTER 5—IDENTIFYING UNCONFESSED SIN

- It disrupts your productivity (Rebekah's actions lacked wisdom).
- It negatively affects the way you treat others (you'll read about Rachel later in this book).
- It reduces your ability to trust in God (even Sarah experienced this phenomenon).

Here is the difference between worry and genuine concern – worry immobilizes, but concern moves you to action. Notice how fear and worry immobilized my friend Gail initially then she turned it into action: *"In 1998 Tim talked about having children again. I said, 'No! I don't want to go through the struggle of trying again.' I prayed to God, 'Lord, could you give me the ability to bear Tim a child without going through the emotional pain again?'*

God's response came through a Bible study I was doing that read: 'I really want to, but if I were to put you into that kind of assignment, you would never be able to handle it. You are just not ready.' So I attended an infertility Bible study group with Christi. Through this group, I was able to let go of the past hurts, but I still struggled with fear of having children. I looked up the word 'fear' in the concordance at the back of my Bible and chose the following four verses to study:

Genesis 26:24 —*'Do not be afraid, for I am with you; I will bless you and will increase the number of your descendants for the sake of my servant Abraham.'*
Psalm 56:3—*'When I am afraid, I will trust you.'*
Matthew 8:26—*'... You of little faith. Why are you afraid?'*
Mark 5:36—*'Don't be afraid, just believe.'*

By admitting and understanding her fears, Gail finally found the courage to return to specialists for further testing. Her doctor's final recommendation was to consider either In Vitro Fertilization or adoption. You will read about the choice Gail and Tim made in Chapter 6.

I would like to add one more thing I learned about fear in my study Bible: *"Planning for tomorrow is time well spent; worrying about tomorrow is time wasted."* I understand that sometimes it's difficult to tell the difference. You probably feel like your life is "on hold" right now. Questions like: *Do we get a big house or a small house? Do we get a 2-door car or a four-door? Should I get a job or go back to school?* are difficult to answer.

Remember, careful planning is thinking ahead about goals, steps, schedules, and trusting in God's guidance. When done well, it can help alleviate worry. The worrier is consumed by fear and finds it difficult to trust God. The worrier lets his plans interfere with his relationship with God. Don't let worries about tomorrow affect your relationship with God today.[12]

Unconfessed Sin and Unanswered Prayer

"If we claim to be without sin, we deceive ourselves and the truth is not in us. If we confess our sins, he is faithful and just and will forgive us our sins and purify us from all unrighteousness. If we claim we have not sinned, we make him out to be a liar and his word has no place in our lives."
1 John 1:8-10

Unconfessed sin results in unanswered prayer and separation from the guidance and protection of Our Heavenly Father. Sometimes I find myself thinking I'm okay with God; I've confessed all of my sins. And then I read the verse above and it makes me stop and think. Right then and there I try to find solitude so I can go to God in prayer and ask Him to reveal anything that might be hindering our relationship – making me unclean before Him. It absolutely amazes me when a flash of memory pops into my head. I try to confess the offense on the spot so I can move on with my life confident that my oneness with Him is in tact.

It is interesting to note how unconfessed sin affected Rachel, wife of Jacob (you will read more about her in Chapter 8). In Genesis 35 you will read that she experienced hard labor and died while giving birth. I find it interesting that she is the only woman the Bible mentions who had hard labor. She had stolen some images of gods from Laban (her father). Jacob wasn't aware of her sin and he made a decree that whomever had stolen them would die. Unconfessed sin caused Rachel's death.

If Christ has forgiven your sins (even the ones you have not committed yet), then why must you confess and repent? Here are four reasons:

1. So that your prayers will not be hindered. First Peter 3:7 says: *"Husbands, in the same way be considerate as you live with your wives, and treat them with respect as the weaker partner and as heirs with you of the gracious gift of life, so that nothing will hinder your prayers."*

CHAPTER 5—IDENTIFYING UNCONFESSED SIN

The reason I bring this verse up is because you are one with your mate and if his prayers are hindered, you will be affected, right? If you are contentious and difficult to live with, you may cause your husband to violate this command and you both will lose out on God's protection and blessings.

Furthermore, verse 12 says: *"For the eyes of the Lord are on the righteous and his ears are attentive to their prayer, but the face of the Lord is against those who do evil."* Most of us don't consider ourselves capable of doing evil, right? Hypothetically speaking, let's say you are angry and feeling resentful toward your partner because he's not as focused on parenthood as you are. You find yourself saying unkind things to him just to get a reaction and your anger graduates into bitterness.

Since this type of scenario occurs in many marriages undergoing infertility, it's time to take a hard look at your self. If you find yourself harboring unconfessed bitterness, anger, pride or resentment, you are allowing evil to prevent God from hearing your prayers. Be cautious!

2. God only listens to the godly man and woman who does his will. In John 9:31(NLT), a blind man who was healed by Jesus said: *"…God doesn't listen to evil men, but he has open ears to those who worship him and do his will."* When most of us think of the word "worship," we generally picture people singing in church, however, the real definition of worship is praising God and living in a fashion that pleases him.

When Pastor Mercer spoke on the subject of worship during our church's 40 Days of Purpose campaign in 2003, he gave three ways to worship God. His thoughts are taken from Pastor Rick Warren of Saddleback Church in Lake Forest, California.[13] They are:

Worship *thoughtfully* by **focusing your attention** on God. How? This is done mostly through prayer; you can worship Him with your thoughts, passions and practices. Think about your words when you pray, give Him quiet time, and pray continually throughout the day.

Worship *passionately* by **expressing your affection to God**. Instead of loving God because of religious duty, show your affection through gratitude, obedience to His Word, by loving Him and worshiping Him and no other God.

Worship *practically* by **using your abilities for God.** Colossians 3:23 reads, ***"Whatever you do, work at it with all your heart, as working for the Lord, not for men…"*** When you go to work, put an honest day's work in. If you're at home doing laundry or ironing clothes, do your best and do it with a good attitude. Make it your goal to please God (2 Corinthians 5:9).

3. Our iniquities separate us from God. *The Living Bible* explains that sin offends God. Because He is holy, He cannot ignore, excuse, or tolerate sin as though it doesn't matter. Sin cuts people off from Him, forming a wall that isolates God from the people He loves (Isaiah 59:2).[14] It seems so simple that He wants us to confess our sins, yet many of us struggle with repentance, humility and pride.

4. The Lord does not hear our prayers (Psalm 66:18). Because we constantly sin, we must constantly ask for forgiveness. Lorie Coleman, author of the Bible study, "Divine Surrender,"[15] defines confession as *"to agree with God that we were wrong."* She says this is true humility. Further, repentance means *"to grieve for sins committed, to feel extreme regret for what one has done or forgotten or omitted to do, to change one's mind and regret the original decision."* She says repentance results in change.

So, how do you avoid sin and make sure your prayers are effective? First, clean up your life. Only you know the "skeletons in your closet." Ask for forgiveness, repent, and forgive yourself or others. Second, stay away from things or people that make you sin. If there are movies or shows on television that aid you in sinful thinking, make sure you're not available when they are on. If you hang out with someone who leads you into sinful areas, let them know that you can no longer participate in such activities. When people say cruel things to you regarding your inability to conceive, be prepared (see Chapter 8) so that you can respond in a righteous manner.

Third, die to sin. For instance, when your mother-in-law calls you on the phone and says, *"So, when are you going to give me a grand baby?"* Instead of sarcastically replying *"When your son's sperm get there act together lady!!"* bite your tongue and in a very compassionate, careful manner, explain you and your husbands plans for adding to your family and any delays that may be occurring. This sounds like a silly example, but anytime our inner self wants to do what we know is wrong, we have to make the choice to do what is right.

I tell you all of this because in your vulnerable state, remember, you are the sheep that Peter refers to in 1 Peter 5:8. The lion desires to single you out; he then crouches and waits for the perfect time to devour you. So, be prepared and aware, be strong and stay with the pack, and use God's strength to fight back.

CHAPTER 5—IDENTIFYING UNCONFESSED SIN

Exposing the Idols of Obsession, Pride and Pity

Idols? Yes, I used the word idols. You're probably thinking I crawled right out of the Old Testament where descriptions of idol worship run rampant. Well, I've got news for you. In this day and age, we've replaced stick carvings and cast gold statues with new idol worship in forms of chemical addictions, sexual promiscuity, self absorption, obsession with beauty, pride, food, recreation, pity, special people in our lives, and other modern-day gods.

Idols are anything that takes the place of God. This is serious business considering the second commandment listed in Exodus 20:4. To remove idols from your life you must recognize their existence and their inability to satisfy you. Stop right where you are reading, and ask God to make you aware of anything unhealthy in your life. He's waiting for you to ask and He will let you know. Once He does, repent of any sin in your life and petition God to help you remove them, so He is the only One who satisfies you.

Satan isn't just playing a little game with you; life is a battlefield, a war to him, and one of his main objectives is to keep you self-focused. Coleman said, *"Prior to the fall of man, Adam and Eve had outward focus. Before Satan could get Adam and Eve to eat the forbidden fruit, he had to work on turning their eyes toward themselves."* She says that once they ate the fruit, *self-focus* occurred and sin was developed. She adds that all Satan has to do is keep you self-focused, and the sins that follow will be automatic.

She goes on to say that Satan uses three strategies to keep self-focus alive in all of us. They are:

Self-Gain (or selfish ambition)— For example, Satan convinced Eve that she needed knowledge in Genesis 3:1-7 and it was a trap. Furthermore, Judas sold out Christ for 30 pieces of silver in Matthew 26:14-16, an ambush by the great deceiver. How does the great deceiver trick you?

Self-Hate (Shame)—Satan uses shame to keep you running from God. The enemy's goal is to take God's healthy conviction to a damaging level of "toxic shame." This keeps unforgiveness (or self disgust) toward your self, alive. She describes "toxic shame" as a thought that makes you re-live something from the past that overwhelms you. The intent is to lead you into depression and spiral you down into suicidal thoughts. To conquer shame, forget the past and look forward – press on toward the prize (which is Christ).

Self-Pity—Coleman says that self-pity is demonic and I agree. She says that it feeds resentment and keeps unforgiveness toward God and others alive. Unforgiveness opens our lives up to demonic influence. For instance, Cain killed his brother Abel (in Genesis 4:1-15), because he was angry and felt sorry for himself.

In her own words, Coleman tells us to *"get a grip!"* and meditate on these verses:

Galatians 2:20—*"I have been crucified with Christ and I no longer live, but Christ lives in me. The life I live in the body, I live by faith in the Son of God, who loved me and gave himself for me."*
Luke 9:23-24—*"...If anyone would come after me, he must deny himself and take up his cross daily and follow me. For whoever wants to save his life will lose it, but whoever loses his life for me will save it."*

We are going to take a closer look at the idols of obsession, pride and pity, however, you may be experiencing other unconfessed sin. As you can see by Sarah's sin, true peace can't exist until you determine any idols in your life, remove them, and allow God to take His rightful place in your life—as number One.

Obsession—A Silent Idol

Satan kept me self-focused by obsession. To say I was fixated with my illusive child seems like an understatement. Every moment of every day I ached for a child. When I was in the car, I pictured a little girl dressed in frilly lace and Mary Jane shoes sitting in the seat next to me. I yearned for her while I was shopping, traveling, and living in general. I craved hearing the word "Mama" from a dependent, little angel. I even woke up each day from eight hours sleep angry that I hadn't been up all night with an infant.

Many women with an only child, not by choice, are so obsessed with creating another child that they miss out on special memories with the first. Time spent studying corrective procedures, testing, and attending doctor's appointments is time spent away from a baby rolling over for the first time or a toddler learning to wave bye-bye.

I refer to obsession as an idol because I had "blind admiration and devotion" to it.[16] *Why is this happening to me?* I would scream. *It hurts too*

CHAPTER 5—IDENTIFYING UNCONFESSED SIN

much to bear Lord, please take away the pain, I begged. In sheer frustration, I wailed, *you said, 'I will not give you more than you can bear' in 1 Corinthians and I'm telling you this is too much!* It felt like I was questioning the Lord and shaking my fist at Him. I reminded Him that Jesus performed miracles, so why couldn't He fix my broken parts.

You have most likely said, felt, or thought this way too. Now that you are aware of the battle going on in your mind, do something about it. Here are some suggestions:

1. Dig deep into the Bible to get to know Christ on a personal basis.
2. Understand that it is okay to ask God what his plans are for you. If the Holy Spirit resides within you, He already knows your thoughts, so it's safe to talk to Him about anything. He says He expects your inquiries and He's anxious to show you His will for your life. James 1:5 says, *"If any of you lacks wisdom, he should ask God, who gives to all without finding fault, and it will be given to him."* Verse six says to be sure to listen for the answers and don't allow yourself to doubt like the double-minded man (or woman in this case).

I have met people who ask everyone's advice on their problems while they need to go to the man in charge instead. Here are four ways the Holy Spirit will usually answer your questions:

Readings from the Bible
Prayer time
Godly people in your life
Circumstances in your life (so be sure to pay attention)

3. Find other women who are walking in your shoes so you will have someone to talk to who understands. If you are unsuccessful, consider studying the ladies I have lovingly labeled the "Bible's Barren Society" closer, or re-read the stories in this book so you feel less lonely.
4. Keep reminding yourself that God DOES have a purpose for your life that will eventually unfold.

I know it's hard to wait, yet you must be patient as you wait for His answers. Remember, they may not always be what you want to hear. Eventually, all of the pieces of the puzzle will come together and make sense.

Pride—Let the Walls Fall Down

There are several forms of pride according to *The American Heritage Dictionary*: 1) Proper and justified self-respect, 2) Pleasure or satisfaction taken in work, achievements, or possessions, and 3) Conceit; arrogance.[17] I am not speaking of these three forms. The pride I refer to is a protective form. I "built shields around myself" by keeping my distance, by pretending that other people's remarks, suggestions and questions didn't hurt me when they actually did, and by bragging that no one would see me cry in public.

Moreover, I continually put on a "mask," or a facade, so I could feel and seem tough. In my family this was good. We weren't "weak" people—we took care of ourselves and we didn't "whine" to others about our problems.

Everywhere I went I wore a great big smile and told everyone I was "just fine." My mask of happiness would go on to force out the gloom. For example, when it was my turn for prayer requests at Bible study, I would pass saying everything was fine in my life. My refusal to ask for prayer was my refusal to admit a problem—all symptoms of pride. Pride is sin. Don't let it become an idol to you.

Look at how Beth Moore defines pride in her Bible study titled "Breaking Free."[18] See if anything sounds familiar to you— it did to me:

- She says that God wants to get to our hearts, but pride covers the heart.
- She adds that God wants to free us from any hindrances in our past, but pride refuses to take a fresh look back.
- God wants to treat us with the prescription of His Word, yet pride doesn't like to be told what to do.
- God wants to set us completely free – pride thinks he's free enough.
- God wants to bring us out of dark closets. Pride says secrets are nobody's business.
- God wants to help us with constraining problems while pride denies there is a problem.
- She concludes that God wants to make us strong in Him, but pride won't admit to weakness.

If your heart didn't sink into your chest with that list, look up these verses:

Proverbs 8:13—God hates pride and arrogance—He considers it evil.
Proverbs 11:2—Pride leads to disgrace—Satan loves disgrace.
Proverbs 13:10—Pride leads to quarrels—Open ground for evil.
Proverbs 16:18—Pride goes before destruction.

CHAPTER 5—IDENTIFYING UNCONFESSED SIN

I fear destruction for anyone, especially you therefore, it is critical that you (and I) make it our goal to practice humility on a moment-to-moment basis. Practice takes commitment, repetition and action. Unfortunately, I wasn't the wisest person and in a sense, I forced God to humble me. After the "act" I described above went on for a while, the "lover of my soul" had enough. He needed to remove the façade, reveal the sin and help me to refocus on Him. He used a dear friend of mine to slap me a wake one day and all the walls I had so carefully built came crumbling down.

This is how He did it: My friends, Lorie and Irene, invited me out to dinner one night. I loved getting out, especially with girlfriends, so I showed up at the restaurant ready for fun. It was not fun. Lorie started out by saying that God puts friends in our lives to bear our burdens with us (Galatians 6:2). She said that by not asking for prayer at Bible study I wasn't allowing my good friends to pray for me, share in my frustration, or even understand the depth of my pain. I started fidgeting in my seat. She continued saying that the mask of happiness I was wearing was pride and that everyone could see right through my act.

She informed me that pride is sin, and that's when I started crying. Conviction hit me right in the gut and I knew she was right. Looking up, I could see patrons staring at me as if they wanted to come to my rescue. I looked for a way of escape and realized I had been set up. Lorie knew me, so she had Irene sit on the outside of the booth so I would be trapped. The more she shared with me, the madder I got. I was so angry I could have slugged her.

Its been around 10 years since that night and I admire Lorie so much for caring enough for me that she put herself through that. She confided in me many years later that she could not sleep the night before and she begged the Lord to have someone else give me that "wake up call." At the time, she seemed mean instead of loving. I look back at that night and see how it was so very necessary and not at all pleasant for her. She was the Lord's *"good and faithful servant."*

Poor, Poor Pitiful Me

The night my friend, Lorie, confronted me, I left that restaurant so angry and upset that I just wanted to find anyone who cared for me and tell them what a meanie she had been. I craved their support and encouragement, but most of all, I wanted their sympathy. The catch is, that wasn't healthy—it's called a pity party. I don't want to sound insensitive, but the "poor, poor pitiful me" attitude is not helpful. It breeds depression, resentment and envy.

The enemy loves pity parties. He's glad to send invitations, decorate, and spin his webs of lies and deception. Pity is his playground and he's no playmate of yours. When you find yourself dealing with low self-esteem and you feel lifeless, remind yourself to capture your thoughts and dispel them. Just picture yourself taking those thoughts and placing them in a balloon and then puncturing the balloon with a pin. Now they are gone and you can fill your mind with healthy, reassuring thoughts. Philippians 4:8 reminds us: *"Finally brothers, whatever is true, whatever is noble, whatever is right, whatever is pure, whatever is lovely, whatever is admirable—if anything is excellent or praiseworthy— think about such things."*

We all experience a degree of self-pity during our journey with infertility. On the other hand, a pity party is when you are so deep into depression that you stay there. It is critical that you realize you are in Satan's grip and that you need to step out of it. Some of the women I have worked with do great for a while and then it's as if they crave the attention they received during their struggle. They revert back to feeling sorry for themselves and swimming in other people's compassion for them. It sounds backwards. This is the epitome of bondage. They not only are in Satan's grip, they are enslaved.

Consider this definition of the word slavery: *"The condition of being a slave; bondage."* Now look at the definition of a slave: *"A person who is owned by and forced to work for someone else. A person completely controlled by a specified influence, emotion, etc."*[19] It should be obvious why pity parties are so dangerous. If you are enslaved to self-pity or someone you care for is, you need to take care of business and eradicate Satan's grip immediately.

How to Fight Back

Now that you are aware that a battlefield surrounds you and that your rival uses sin, self-focus and idols to war against you, be prepared to fight back. I've already told you how. The Armor of God which is defined in Ephesians 6:11-17 is your weapon. Get to know what God says, memorize verses to help you fight off the evil one, and then use those verses *against him*. You see, since Satan is literally the father of lies, he can't stand in the truth—he has to flee *("Submit yourselves, then, to God. Resist the devil, and he will flee from you." James 4:7)*

CHAPTER 5—IDENTIFYING UNCONFESSED SIN

When you feel him in your presence, use the Bible to rebuke him by saying out loud *"Satan, you have no authority over me. I belong to Jesus and his blood has washed away my sins. In the name of Jesus Christ and by the authority of the truth, I command you to flee from me just like James 4:7 says,"* and he will.

If you are wondering how Satan knows God's Word, remember that before his displacement from heaven, he was an archangel. He knows God well; he once adored our Lord. He knows the Bible backward and forward. But, get this – he is very familiar with Revelation 20:10(NLT): *"Then the devil who had betrayed them will again be thrown into the Lake of Fire burning with sulphur where the Creature and False Prophet are, and they will be tormented day and night forever and ever."*

With that in mind, remember that he wants to keep the trial of infertility from strengthening your spiritual walk. Because of your vulnerability, he will try to seduce you into spending *your* future on "his side." Just use this verse to remind him of *his* future!

Next, practice obedience. When I was a child, I was obedient because I wanted to please my parents. I couldn't stand the idea of disappointing them. Obedience to God is basically the same. It is a desire to please the Lord with the way you choose to live your life. Choices are made everyday. You can choose to wake up grumpy or you can wake up in the morning and thank God for the miracle of the sunrise. You can choose to listen to idle gossip, or you can walk away. You choose to be Christ-like by avoiding situations or people who lead you into temptation.

For instance, Susan and her husband experienced great difficulties during their journey. It seemed like the enemy tried to trip them up everywhere they turned; however they kept their faith. They chose obedience and they were rewarded in the end: *"My first miscarriage occurred at three months during our first pregnancy,"* said Susan. *"I was going in for my first ultrasound to see if we could hear a heartbeat. The doctor kept looking and didn't say anything. It went on and on. She could not detect a heartbeat and so she sent me to the hospital.*

My heart sank as the second ultrasound confirmed that the baby had died. We endured the heartbreak of a D&C (this procedure is described in Chapter 9) unaware of the road of emotions and physical/spiritual struggles the Lord was preparing us to travel.

A year later we were unsuccessfully able to conceive on Clomid, so we tried intrauterine insemination (IUI) with my husband's sperm. I had three eggs that month *(with Clomid) and amazingly God allowed us to conceive our daughter. Every time I went to the bathroom I was afraid of finding blood, but I didn't and on my 30th birthday, my precious angel was born – healthy and wonderful!"*

Susan was relieved that the trial of infertility was over, but the next trial began when her baby girl was 15 months old— Susan's husband was diagnosed with testicular cancer. *"We were encouraged to 'bank' some sperm because chemotherapy would damage what was left leaving him sterile afterward. To be honest, we were more concerned with his health at that point than potential infertility, but with the encouragement of family, we did bank four specimens.*

After 1 1/2 years, he was doing fine, and we decided to use one of the specimens and try IUI again. The day I started my period, my husband told me he was having symptoms again, this time on the other side. I was devastated when we learned he had cancer—a new case they said—and we would be going through all of it again. But again, God knew the limits of our strength," Susan said.

"We helped start 'Living Courageously'—a cancer-support group through our church. Their encouragement, love and focus on Christ's strength got us through many a weary day. We felt so blessed to have our daughter, but as my husband recovered, I began to long for more children. My husband felt sad and angry at times because he was no longer able to 'give' me children, although I never ever thought for one second that it was his fault, Susan recalls.

Through amazing generosity and miracles, funding was secured so that Susan and her husband could undergo In Vitro Fertilization three times. Unfortunately, Susan's ovaries didn't respond well to the required fertility drugs and she ended up wrestling with secondary infertility.

On their third attempt Susan conceived! I remember the joyous celebrations of so many people in our community and then the great disappointment when she miscarried six weeks later. It seemed that all of her chances for more little feet running through her house were gone. So many of us were so confused – we wondered why God allowed all of this to happen, but Susan did the right thing. She ran to her Bible and she claimed this verse: Romans 8:28— *"And we know that in all things God works for the good of those who love him, who have been called according to his purpose."*

When we would get together, she would remind me that He had a bigger plan. I remember her saying, *"He is calling me to trust Him. That is one of the hardest lessons I'm learning—trust. He knows what is best. He loves me. He never takes His eyes off me."*

Because I was still dealing with my own infertility issues, I had so much

CHAPTER 5—IDENTIFYING UNCONFESSED SIN

respect for my friend and her family. Year after year went by as I witnessed her struggling, yet I also saw her faith growing and it was contagious. I watched and I waited. I wasn't aware of it, but apparently Susan's husband was against adoption. She revealed to me recently that his exact words had been: *"If God wants us to have another child, He will drop one in our laps!"*

Susan recalls her feelings: *"For years I battled with desire, guilt and frustration. Our little girl prayed every night that Jesus would bring her a little baby brother or sister! I wanted to tell her, 'Stop praying that, don't you realize God said NO!' When she turned eight I really had come to a place of peace about our family size. It didn't even bother me anymore when others told me the news of their expanding families.*

Then on one cold November night, God did exactly what He'd planned all along, He 'Plopped' a baby in our laps. We now have an adopted, fabulous daughter—the sister my little girl prayed for. And if we hadn't gone through infertility and cancer, we wouldn't have learned to trust, and ultimately, we would have lost out on such a precious gift.

My husband adores her just as much as our first child. She has added a new dimension to our family and so much joy to our lives. Amazingly, both our hearts are open to any other children the Lord chooses to drop in our laps!"

Last, learn a valuable lesson from Susan: instead of hiding from Satan and fearing that he's lurking around every corner, hold tight to your faith. Colossians 1:13, 14 (NLT) reminds us that *"he has rescued us out of the darkness and gloom of Satan's kingdom and brought us into the Kingdom of his dear Son, who bought our freedom with his blood and forgave us all of our sins."* Work through this time of growth and focus on Christ. The evil one won't feel invited back once he witnesses your devotion to God and your faith in His plans for your family.

I'll be Strong and Hold on Tight

Infertility is not a common word to say.
Most people don't use it everyday.
Only those who share this challenge of ours,
Can realize the anguish and sadness it bears.

It hurts so much, you're aching inside.
You put up a front, but how can you hide?
You see pregnant ladies walking the mall,
Newborns in strollers, toddlers who fall.

Now you can hardly hold back the tears.
It's there, it's tugging, all of the fears.
When, oh when, will this pain go away?
No one really knows – it's hard to say.

For now I'll be strong and hold on real tight,
I'll keep all my hopes and try not to lose sight.
For only God knows what His plan is for me.
It may not be what I think it will be.

We may or may not have a birthchild of our own,
But through this experience I have truly grown!
I don't know how this journey of faith will end,
Lord, teach me contentment in whatever you send.

By Nancy A. Ely-Morse[20]

"You, dear children, are from God and have overcome them, because the one who is in you is greater than the one who is in the world."
1 John 4:4

Chapter Six–Surrendering Your Plans

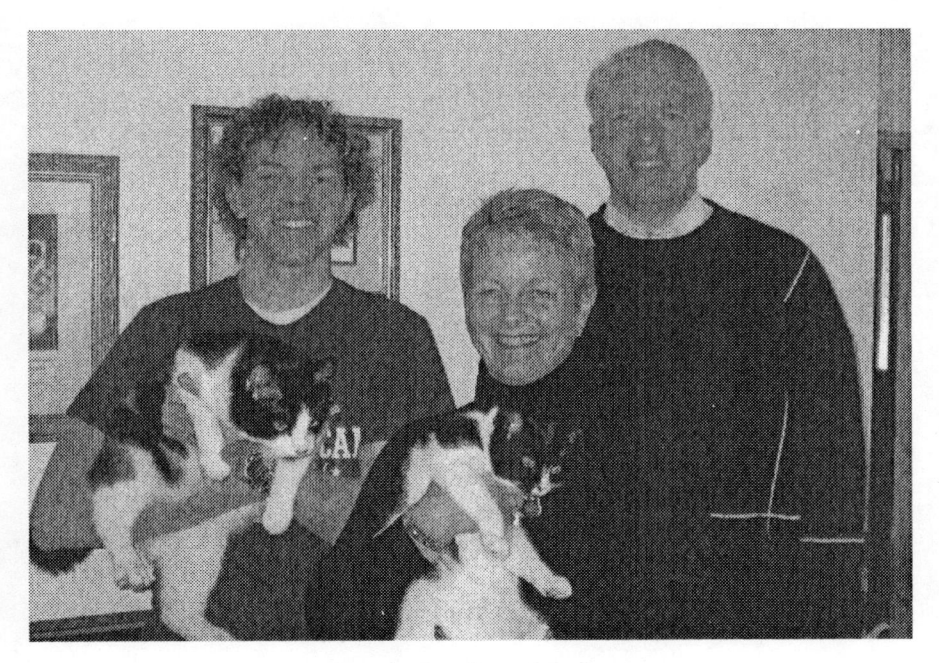

Doug, Ruth and Dale

-Surrendering Your Will For God's Will
    How to Surrender
-Waiting on God's Perfect Timing
    What Happens When You Choose Not to Surrender

Chapter Six–Surrendering Your Plans

1. What do you think of when I say you must "surrender your will?" (Giving up your Last Will and Testament? Becoming a "doormat" for others to walk on? Giving up your rights? Being crushed by God? Experiencing God's perfect plan for your life?)

_____
_____
_____

2. Have you ever been labeled a "control freak?" Yes or No?

3. Do you feel angry at the unfairness of infertility or are you angry with God for letting this happen to you?

_____
_____
_____

4. Have you felt the urge to "help God" bring a child into your home? Yes or No? If so, what were the circumstances? Please explain:

_____
_____
_____

5. Have you set a time line for pregnancy or a date you *have* to have a baby by? Yes or No? If yes, write it here:

_____

_____

_____

6. Go up to question #5 and erase or cross out your date – for good!

7. List five ways you can practice patience during this difficult time:
    1)_____
    2)_____
    3)_____
    4)_____
    5)_____

8. Do you believe God may be "timing" your conception like He did with Elizabeth, the mother of John the Baptist? Yes or No? Can you handle it if God makes it clear that He wants you to move on as a complete family? Yes or No?

9. What do you believe could happen if you choose to "have it your way" rather than surrendering to God's will and His timing?

_____

_____

_____

Recommended Reading:

Proverbs 3:5-6   Isaiah 55:9
Matthew 6:7-15, 10:32-33   Luke 9:23-25

CHAPTER 6—SURRENDURING YOUR PLANS

Romans 6:1-13, 15-18, 12:1, 2
Galatians 2:20, 5:16-18
Philippians 3:8, 9, 4:19
Hebrews 4:13
2 Corinthians 12:9
Ephesians 1:17-18
Colossians 2:13-15
James 4:13-16

Look up these verses and fill in the blanks:

James 1:2-4 (NLT): *"Dear brothers, is your life full of difficulties and temptations? Then be happy, for when the way is rough, your patience has a chance to _____. So let it grow, and don't try to squirm out of your problems. For when your patience is finally in full bloom, then you will be ready for anything, strong in character, full and _____."*

1 Peter 3:17 (TRSV): *"For it's better to suffer for doing right, if that should be God's _____, then for doing wrong."*

Mark 8:34-35 (NLT): *"Then he called his disciples and the crowds to come over and listen. 'If any of you wants to be my follower,' he told them, 'you must put aside your own pleasures and shoulder your cross, and follow me closely. If you insist on saving your life, you will _____ it. Only those who throw away their lives for my sake and for the sake of the Good News will ever know what it means to really _____.'"*

"Why do I Have to Wait so Long?"
Answer #5—A barren womb teaches you to surrender your will and your timing for God's perfect will and His timing

Chapter 6—Elizabeth's Story

My name is Elizabeth and for many years I lived as an outcast. Because I was aged and childless, I faced public shame and loneliness in Judea. My husband, Zacharias, and I suffered social ridicule and hopelessness – the people in our land actually considered us "cursed." It would have been permissible back then for Zach to create a child for me with my maidservant, but we decided to move on as a family of two.

Zacharias traveled often to the Temple in Jerusalem to perform his priestly duties leaving me home alone with my torment. Simple things like my daily walk to the well were as devastating as a modern-day woman's trip to the mall. I faced finger pointing, thoughtless comments, ridicule and constant reminders of my empty arms at such an old age. Yet my faith in the Lord remained steady.

One day my life changed forever—Zach returned from the Temple and he was so excited, he could hardly breathe. A dream I had long ago given up on was about to come true. Zacharias announced that I was going to have a baby! An angel told my husband that God had heard his prayers and that he would bless us with a son, whom we were to name John. He was to be one of the Lord's great men. I was astonished and aghast with joy. But that's not the end of the story.

A few days after I learned I would give birth, my niece, Mary, who lived 70 miles north of here in Nazareth, learned from an angel that she too would become pregnant with Christ, the Messiah. The way I saw it, four miracles were happening at once: 1) An old, barren woman would conceive, 2) a young virgin would bear a child, 3) the Savior of the world was to be born soon, and 4) the Lord had timed my pregnancy so that my son (who later was known as John the Baptist), would be the messenger for Christ.[1]

> **"What an honor this is, that the mother of my Lord should visit me! When you came in and greeted me, the instant I heard your voice, my baby moved in me for joy! You believed that God would do what he said; that is why he has given you this wonderful blessing." Luke 1:43-45 (NLT)**

Surrendering Your Will for God's Will

I have talked about surrender throughout this book and to define it as clearly as possible, I will use the analogy of a wild horse. During my long journey, I kicked and bucked and stomped and snorted my way through frustration, anger, and anxiety. God waited patiently. He didn't force Himself on me. He didn't bridle me or beat me. He knew I was restless and wanted to run free instead of being caged in and controlled. So, He basically waited until I wore myself out. Instead of "breaking me," He wisely let me break myself. When I was finally broken, it was by my own doing.

Are you in a place where this sounds familiar? Have you ever witnessed someone hitting rock bottom? It's not pleasant, however, once they do, they are finally rational. That's where I was. I finally gave up and relinquished control of my plans and said, *"Okay God! Do what you're going to do because what I'm doing isn't working."* Not everyone who experiences infertility goes through this unpleasant exercise. Hopefully you will learn from my tantrums and make better choices.

After witnessing many women's reactions to infertility, I noticed that each one went through stages or processes. In 1969, Dr. Elisabeth Kubler-Ross wrote the book, *On Death and Dying.*[2] In it, she pioneered the Five Stages of Grief. I have added my own little twist to her research and believe these are five stages you will experience as you grieve the the bewilderment of barrenness:

Shock/Denial
Anger/Obsession
Bargaining/Desperation
Depression/Mourning
Acceptance or Bitterness

Knowing these stages are going to occur should make it easier for you to know what to expect. You'll realize the reactions you experience are normal and healthy. They may not occur in order—you might feel deep sorrow one moment then incredible anger the next, only to find yourself completely detached afterwards.

You may be thinking that only the readers who experience miscarriage or loss will go through these stages, yet look back and see from the various testimonies how even ladies with primary and secondary infertility experienced them as well. For instance, we all undergo a level of **shock** once we learn a child may not be part of our family unit. Some women such as Gail and I **deny** problems and instead of putting faith into action, we wait around wasting valuable time.

Anger is normal when everyone around you seems to go on with their lives leaving you stranded and stagnant. This is especially true for women who have undergone miscarriage and it seems like the subject is "taboo."

It's easy to focus strictly on what you've been robbed of, hence **obsession** becomes predominant. A great example of this phenomenon occured when Rachel was so jealous of her sister Leah's ability to reproduce that she became obsessed with competing in a child bearing race. (You will read about this in Chapter 8.)

Once we've settled down and started looking at different options such as testing, advanced testing, adoption and fostering, some women fall into the **bargaining** trap. You will read in Chapter 10 how a lady named Mary told the Lord she would give up caffeine beverages if he would just fulfill her dream of motherhood. Another example of bargaining includes walking into an adoption agency with a pre-established list of conditions (such as we don't want an open adoption, we've decided against twins or sibling sets) and then crumbling when the mention of an available child comes up.

At some point the majority of us become **desperate.** We'll do anything to show the Lord and the world that we mean business and we'll do anything necessary to facilitate childbirth. Sarah did, didn't she? She was so desperate for an heir that she actually arranged for her husband, Abraham, to sleep with another woman!

Depression is an expected stage of grieving (especially for mothers who lost their babies) because they and the barren are in a stagnant state. We have a loss and we don't know how to handle it. We can't control our future... we can't make plans...we don't fit in anymore. This reminds me of Hannah who became so depressed that she couldn't even eat! This stage is normal and I advise you to pay attention to your surroundings. Just make sure to grieve and mourn so you get it out of your system, but watch that the enemy doesn't lead you into a deep, dark hole that you can't crawl out of.

Mourning occurs as you grieve the loss. This period may last a long time for some women which is natural. As you cry, the sorrow, distress, sadness and anguish are released from your body. This is important. If you try to stuff those feelings down deep inside, your body will experience physical discomfort, plus you will eventually explode emotionally one day.

Hopefully you will allow yourself to undergo these stages naturally so that **bitterness** doesn't set in. If you think mourning is a dark period, realize that bitterness is even bleaker. It will negatively affect all areas of your life: your friendships, your marriage, your career and your relationship with God. On the otherhand, **acceptance**, which I equate with surrender, is such a better way to live.

Lisa surrendered to the Lord in a letter she wrote to Him: "*Oh, how good it feels when, to my amazement, I learn that I'm expecting my second child. I vow to take good care of myself. No longer do I have to look at all those pregnant women with longing. I'm one of them! And then I wake up and find out that this was only a dream. The same old feelings of anger, futility, depression, and hopelessness wash over me, just as they do when I begin my period every month. I realize that, in my particular financial and family situation, medical treatments are inaccessible and adoption isn't an option. Why can't I take what seems to be your firm 'No!' for an answer?"*[3]

She ends the letter by saying: *"Please deliver me from this non-stop yearning. Help me as I grieve for the large, stable, Christian family I will never have. In its place, please give me more of you, and, in other ways, fill my life with blessings. I put this matter in your hands, for I know that you can do miracles and that your plan is for our good."* Surrender is never easy, but look at how much calmer she seemed once she handed this huge issue over to her Heavenly Father.

Susan learned about surrender through the wisdom of her sister: *"I can remember distinctly having a telephone conversation with my sister about my inability to conceive. I told her 'I won't be able to handle it if God never allows me to be a mom!' Her response was God's seed that began my complete surrender. She said, 'Well, you'll never be a mom until you're okay with not being one.'"*

How to Surrender

Coleman put a lot of thought into the issue of surrender when she wrote her Bible study therefore, I will be sharing many of her teachings with you. She says there are two major decisions you need to make in order to tap into the abundant life Jesus made available (John 10:10).

She says the first step is accepting Christ as your personal Savior. She says it is the easiest decision you will ever make. *"It doesn't take any work on your part – you just open your heart and receive the greatest free gift ever. It's that easy!"* Coleman says the second decision you must make is to "give your life to Christ." She adds, *"Through the first decision, we easily receive; through the second decision, we painfully give.*

Some people do accept Christ as their Savior and surrender their lives to Him at the same time, but I believe it is rare," she says. *"It is more common to receive Jesus and have several years go by before you realize that you also need to give Him control of your life. And even after you realize that you need to give Him your life, it can be even longer before you truly make that decision! The sad truth is that there are many, many Christians who die without ever giving God their lives—they only received the free gift [of salvation]."*

Coleman suggests three steps to surrender. They are:

1. Give up your will—She says, *"Although I believe the second decision, surrendering your life to Christ, is a one-time decision, it does occur in steps and requires daily upkeep. The first step to surrender is giving up your will. This is where the fight with God stops over who will have control of your life.*

Before I reached this point in my spiritual life, I had been trying to live my life my own way for quite a while. I had reached the conclusion that my way wasn't working. I had made a mess of my life already. That is when the white flag went up, the towel was thrown into the ring, and my will was ready to admit defeat and surrender. This is when the 'Whatever, God' prayer of surrender was made: whatever He chose to do with me and my circumstances, I would accept, and whatever He commanded me, I would obey. Throwing up my hands and releasing my present circumstances and attitudes was the most difficult, yet freeing thing I ever did. Only at this step is God able to tame the heart of a man or woman."

2. Give up your rights—She continues, *"The second step in the surrender process is to give up the rights to yourself. This is another area where many Christians are stunted in their growth. Just as the will says, 'I want,' our self rights say, 'I deserve!' My flesh has always demanded the rights to myself and to satisfy my every desire. This is where I had to make the choice to abandon myself and run to God. The person I wanted to leave most in life was myself anyway, so I emotionally left me. I left all of my selfish desires mixed with unrealistic expectations and ran to God. I ran to Him like a prisoner set free, threw myself before His throne, and yielded myself to His rules and desires. I no longer trusted my life to me. I gave Him my rights, my life, and my body to use as He pleased."*

3. Give up your image— *"As my will says, 'I want,' and my rights say, 'I deserve,' my image asks, 'what will people think?' My image comes down to pride, because, in every case, pride is what nourishes the image."* Coleman says there are two kinds of people who are worried about what others think: One, new Christians who are truly living for Christ. They are being drawn in by the love of Jesus and the realization that they need Him. She says the fear of giving Him control of their life is that others will see a change in them, and that's embarrassing.

"There may even be the concern of losing loved ones over this choice. However, in Matthew 10:33, Jesus draws the line in the sand for those who wish to move forward in their relationship with Him when He says, 'But

CHAPTER 6—SURRENDURING YOUR PLANS

whoever shall deny Me before men, I will also deny him before My Father who is in heaven.' True, this step in the surrender process can seem risky, and you may suffer some loss, but it is very necessary. God never allows you to give up more than He gives back.

The second kind of Christian who worries about what others think is, in my terminology, *'wearing a mask.'* This is where the problem begins for many *'churched'* people. They are very willing to give their time in reading the Bible, praying, church attendance, tithing, and serving in ministries, but they want to keep control of their image! In other words, they don't want others to see any flaws in them," she concludes.

When you go through this process, you may want to journal your thoughts or even write a letter to God like Lisa did in the previous section. Some people place their letters in a secret place and read them at a future date, others write the letter and then burn it—you decide what will be the most comforting for you.

Another way to release pent-up emotions and burdens is to have what Coleman labeled a "gut wrencher." I am confident that anyone enduring the disappointments of infertility will benefit from this exercise. Here are the seven steps Coleman advises:

1. Make sure you are going to be alone or will not be bothered for a length of time. Take the phone off the hook or let the answering machine take messages.

2. Get in the most humble position for you. Some people are flat on the ground, some lie on their back. Others are on their knees with their face to the ground. Whatever is most humbling to you – do it!

3. Pour out your heart to God. This is the time to scream, yell, cry and complain about your pain to God. If you say to yourself, 'I can't complain to God,' then I ask you, if God lives in you, doesn't He already know how you feel? Why lie about how you feel? He is waiting to deal with the problem if you will just come to Him honestly.

4. Ask Him to forgive you for every fault that comes to your mind that you personally are guilty of in the situation... WITH NO BUT's! (i.e. I'm sorry I was jealous, but...) This is good practice for when we stand before the great white throne of God and have to answer for our own actions without blaming others for what we have done.

5. Release your rights if you feel you have been innocent and the circumstances haven't been fair to you. Accept your discipline if you have been wrong (without excuses). Give God the problem and leave it with Him! Picture yourself before His throne laying down a package and then walking away. Don't go back and pick it up!

6. Thank Him for taking the burden and ask Him to protect your heart and mind while He solves the problem His way.

7. Don't leave God's presence until you feel the release of your burden.

I believe nothing gets past God—especially our burdens. Hebrews 4:13 reads *"Nothing in all creation is hidden from God's sight. Everything is uncovered and laid bare before the eyes of him to whom we must give account."* He knows your hurts and disappointments. He knows this trial will make you stronger. All He asks is that you trust Him with the life *He* gave you.

Waiting on God's Perfect Timing

Nobody likes to wait. If we're driving, we take the fast lane, if we're cooking, we use the microwave, and if we're shopping, we head for the shortest check-out line.

My friend, Charlene, is no different. Read how she set her own timeline for pregnancy without first considering God's plans. Once she decided she wanted a baby, she immediately formulated a plan: *"I told my mildly surprised husband to put away the condoms. We'd be pregnant by late October, but we'd wait until Christmas to tell the rest of the family. When I got my period in October I figured we just hadn't started early enough in my cycle to conceive.*

So, I put my husband on notice that we were going into battle and that he should prepare himself for lots of sex. We would be sending a daily armada of sperm in to shower friendly fire on the elusive egg. Imagine our surprise in November when I got my period again. I didn't get concerned until December when I was still not pregnant.

As previously planned, we had the whole family over for the holiday. Instead of announcing my good news to the family, my brother and his wife, who had only been married for two months, announced their baby was due in July. My family celebrated around the Christmas tree. I went to my bedroom and cried."

We are all human—we set timetables, we make demands and we occasionally give up on God. Even Elizabeth, who was a very godly woman,

CHAPTER 6—SURRENDURING YOUR PLANS

seems to have given up on having a child. She was probably shocked beyond belief when Zacharias made the announcement that she would soon be a mother. She waited on the Lord and in turn, he *timed* the birth of her son and blessed her for her patience. No matter how impossible God's promises seem, He always keeps them, probably not the very next day, but at the proper time.

Eileen speaks to barren Christian women at conferences and she says that having patience and accepting God's will are the issues that trip most of us up. She says, *"There is no doubt that scripturally God created us male and female for the purpose of procreation within the confines of marriage. So, as I always say, God does not command us to go out and be fruitful and multiply only to set us up for failure."*

She says that most women (and their husbands) need to clean house spiritually first. She says that everyone seems to skip around the issues of healing and deliverence. Eileen explains, *"Past sexual sin even affected future generations in the Bible. One needs to earnesly seek God for answers. I believe that He will give us the answers in His time. Perseverence is also an issue. There are many ladies I know who did not conceive until they were married for over 20 years. Why should we think that Sarah and Elizabeth were to be the only old ladies having children?*

All too often I see people give up hope. They just move on to adoption as a quick fix to saving themselve future heartache, while God could be using that difficult time to perfect them in some way. I am not trying to bash adoption if that is where someone really believes God is leading them in prayer, yet I see the level of humility not being where it should be. Why aren't people waiting on God?" she asks.

God planned our lives before He created the universe, therefore, sometimes His timing and ours don't coincide. Sometimes we pray and pray for something good and upright only for Him to withhold his answer for a while. God has reasons for unanswered prayer; I can only speculate what they might be:

-God deepening our insight into what we really need.
-God broadening our appreciation for His answers.
-God allowing us to mature so we can use His gifts more wisely.
-Our request does not fall in line with His plans for us.
-Our request does not fall in line with His timing and we need to wait.
-Due to unconfessed sin, our prayers are hindered.

Do you recall Abraham and Sarah's story? Their situation seemed impossible too; I sympathize with Sarah and can appreciate why she grew impatient and took matters into her own hands. I was tempted many times to "help God." I remember receiving so many phone calls from well-meaning people who knew of a situation where a child needed a home. One involved a friend who knew the mother of a young girl looking for a home for her unborn baby; another was a married couple that decided they would seek adoption for their child after its birth. I recall hanging up the phone each time jubilantly asking the Lord "is this the one?"

I would get myself all worked up and begin to feel the desire to help the Lord out. I told him I'd be happy to help out by making some phone calls or perhaps meeting those people, and one by one, each scenario fell through. After a year of turmoil I finally wised up and learned to wait on the Lord. It wasn't easy at first, but it sure beat giving myself an ulcer!

Be careful when you are in these positions. You must ascertain whether God is showing you the road to take or if Satan is distracting you from where your focus should be.

It can be difficult to be patient during these periods. This is how David described patience and waiting on God in Psalm 40:1-4 (NLT)—*"I waited patiently for God to help me; then he listened and heard my cry. He lifted me out of the pit of despair, out from the bog and mire, and set my feet on a hard, firm path and steadied me as I walked along.*

He has given me a new song to sing, of praises to our God. Now many will hear of the glorious things he did for me, and stand in awe before the Lord, and put their trust in him. Many blessings are given to those who trust the Lord, and have no confidence in those who are proud, or who trust in idols."

David says he "waited patiently." On question number seven I asked you to list some ways you can practice patience during this difficult time. Go back and look at your answers. Frankly, your patience may be worn thin by now, so I've jotted down some ideas I hope you will add to your list:

1. Keep reading and praying daily.
2. Continue intensifying your relationship with the Lord and getting to know Him better (Bible studies have really helped me).
3. Do not allow yourself to give up on God or yourself.
4. If you are waiting during the adoption process, don't expect yourself to just forget your desire for pregnancy overnight.
5. Be patient with yourself as you *learn* to trust God more and more daily.

It takes time.

6. Consider a time-consuming hobby or short-term job. Having a job while I waited to adopt helped keep my mind off of "the wait."

7. Do not acquaint yourself with people or things that bend toward pity parties or temptation to sin.

8. Purposely search for things to be grateful for and then shout to the heavens with gratitude. Feeling thankful will help alleviate the blues.

9. Be yourself. Be confident in who you are. Consider releasing your secret to selected family and friends and never consider yourself broken, inadequate, or undesirable.

10. Make your marriage a priority (I have specific suggestions in Chapter 10).

11. If you are experiencing secondary infertility, spend quality time with your family. Realize you can't bury your desire for an expanded family overnight.

12. Consider counseling from a therapist or pastor if you need encouragement and support.

13. Pamper yourself.

14. Meditate on 2 Corinthians 12:9: "*...My grace is sufficient for you, for my power is made perfect in weakness.*'" Basically Jesus was telling Paul, and therefore all of us, that we aren't supposed to know everything. He exhorts us to let His grace and His power be enough.

15. Rekindle any relationships that may have been neglected or negatively affected during the journey.

16. Remind yourself that God is the maker of miracles.

Speaking of miracles, do you remember Gail? Her first husband divorced her because of infertility; she searched for answers for 10 years; her second husband wanted children; and she struggled with fear. Here's the rest of her story:

"*I finally came to a point in my life when I could accept the fact that I was not going to have children and adoption may be the only way. I remember reading, 'God wants you to depend on Him—not a method or a program.' We have completed the adoption process and are now waiting patiently to adopt. God is in control—we are depending on Him to provide us with the child perfect for our family.*

I still go through times when I think I can get pregnant. Then I find out that someone else is pregnant the day I start my period. Those are the toughest days for me. I thank God that I have been able to handle my emotions through this second attempt to have children. I am really trusting God to make the final decision on which child will be with us."

Last, surrendering your timing for God's is a *decision*, it is an *attitude* and it has *great results*. Allow me to break this down for you:

Surrender is a Decision—I was beginning to give up on Gail. I've known her for around eight years and even though we talked about surrender so many times, I just didn't see evidence of it. She seemed dead set on getting pregnant and her fear of adoption was great.

Her fears about loving someone else's child and what would happen if she didn't bond with an adopted child made me uneasy. I felt her fears were too much to overcome and her opposition to any form of contact with the birth parents was based on a great deal of apprehension.

Last week Gail called me and said a birth mother had chosen them to parent her unborn baby. She proceeded to tell me the birth mother lives down the street, attends the same church and wants to interact with the baby even in the capacity of babysitting. I was floored that Gail would even consider this. I was amazed at the confidence and peace in her voice. There was a brand new person on the other end of the phone—a surrendered woman, not a desperate one.

It hit me that I had given up on her, but God hadn't. He chose this child for her to mother and he had used a great deal of time to get her to the point of surrender. A miracle took place right in front of my eyes! She and her husband are now the very proud parents of a son! That's so cool!

Surrender is an Attitude—In Philippians 3:8-9, Paul says, *"What is more, I consider everything a loss compared to the surpassing greatness of knowing Christ Jesus my Lord, for whose sake I have lost all things. I consider them rubbish, that I may gain Christ and be found in him, not having a righteousness of my own that comes from the law, but that which is through faith in Christ—the righteousness that comes from God and is by faith."*

Paul considered all of his accomplishments rubbish (defined as *something discarded as trash*). [4] He gave up everything—his family, friendships, and political freedom in order to know Christ and his resurrection power. I'm not asking you to do that however, this attitude of unselfishness will help you make needed sacrifices.

Romans 12:1 tells us to offer our bodies as living sacrifices, holy and pleasing to God. Paul tells us this is our spiritual act of worship. Coleman hit on this when she talked about giving up your will. To offer your bodies as living sacrifices means to lay aside your own desires and follow Him.

For example, when a friend of mine had her endometrial biopsy she screamed at the pain. Her doctor asked, *"Oh, did that hurt?"* She wanted to blurt out, *"let's stick a needle in your scrotum and see if that hurts mister!"* but she calmed herself instead and was cordial to him. It may sound silly, but that's an example of my friend "dying to herself."

Anytime we do the right thing, or hold our tongue, or refrain from hurting others, we are dying to our own selfish desires. Another example would include finding an alternative to pornography when your husband has to "do his business" in the cup. Yes, he has to ejaculate to make this happen, but he should be thinking of you, not another woman.

Surrender has Great Results—Mary tried to conceive for four years. Look at the great results she experienced after her surrender: "*I remember the first year was not too bad; I told myself it took some couples that long. As the first year turned to the second, and then the third, a sense of desperation overshadowed me. Often during those four years I read Hannah's story in 1 Samuel 1. I didn't feel quite as alone or guilty when I learned that Hannah had bitterness of soul (verse 10). Oh, how I could relate to that!*

The following January, after surviving a grueling Christmas and feeling especially down, I took out my Bible once again, and cried to God for grace and strength. 1 Samuel 1:13-16 and 18 leaped out of the pages at me. I read those verses and prayed with tears streaming down my face. Hannah, in verse 18, gave it all to God and was no longer downcast. After I, too, gave it all to God and told Him to show me what road to take next, I felt a sense of love, grace and compassion."[5]

You may desire to control your future, but it's like trying to harness the ocean—it's impossible. Many of us are control freaks—it's our nature, but moving on with your life and acquiring freedom from this burden requires surrender.

What Happens When You Choose Not to Surrender

God gave us free will. He could have made us all puppets that did whatever He said, when He said to do it. Instead, He teaches us to make good choices. What happens if you decide against surrendering your will for God's? (This can even happen subconsciously.) I certainly don't have all the answers, although I have witnessed this phenomenon. This is what could possibly happen in my opinion:

Nothing —Do it your way and nothing might happen. What does that mean? It means more waiting. What does more waiting bring about? More frustration, more anguish and more disappointment. Does this sound fun? Absolutely not – it sounds unbearable.

Disappointment—I know of a woman who was dead-set on helping God find her little girl. She was one of those Christians who seemed very "spiritual" on the outside, yet her controlling nature wasn't very attractive. She found a young pregnant girl quite literally on a street corner and invited her to live in her home until the baby was born (without overtly praying for God's guidance in the matter).

Once the baby was born, she was quick to show off her beautiful, new, baby girl just like any of us would do. Two years later that little girl developed a fatal disease. You might be thinking this mother was punished – hold on, I disagree. Perhaps God knew this sweet child would only spend two years on this earth and he intended for this woman to mother a different child. Perhaps she "jumped the gun" and paid a great price.

Loss of Protection—Another woman I know lived a secret life. She used infertility as a disguise. While people were focusing on the struggle she was going through, she was sinning in other areas unbeknownst to them. I witnessed many bad decisions on her part and because she was aware of these poor choices, God could no longer protect her. She came dangerously close to losing her marriage, family and freedom.

Loss of Blessings—If you beg the Lord for a baby for years and years, do not make the mistake of putting limits or conditions on your prayers. One lady I counseled wanted a baby girl for years. She was so in love with this baby girl that existed in her mind, that she was consumed with finding her. It seemed like she was unable to enjoy life and any inkling of happiness with the family she had until she had "her little Angela."

Finally when a birth mother chose her to mother her child, she told the agency "no" because the mother was unsure if the baby was a girl. Things went from bad to worse until she finally gave up the struggle and opened her arms to what *God* had in store for her. She has a baby girl now and interestingly enough her name is Victoria.

Marital Problems—Since you are "one" with your husband, that means your bad decisions will more than likely affect him, right? Let's say you force him to adopt when he has made it clear that he is ready to call it quits and continue life *without* children. *If* you successfully adopt, do you think he'll be a great father to "someone else's child?" Do you think there might be friction when you expect him to spend time with the baby, especially when you really need a break? What kind of marriage and family life would that create? A sad existence and possibly a breakup when that child needs a solid home.

Bitterness—Bitterness is defined as: *"Exhibiting or proceeding from strong animosity ('bitter hostility or hatred'). Having or marked by resentfulness or disappointment."*[6] In her Bible Study, "A Woman's Heart, God's Dwelling Place,"[7] Beth Moore refers to bitterness as "spiritual cancer." She says it cannot be ignored, but must be healed at the very core and only Christ can heal it. She adds that no one can do it for you and no one can tell you exacly what is required for your healing. Others can direct you to Jesus, but you must show up for your appointments. His ultimate goal is not simply for you to be healed but for you to meet the Healer.

It seems obvious why the enemy loves bitterness – it keeps your eyes on yourself and your past – not on God. Bitterness keeps you looking in the rear view mirror and if you hold on to it, you will not be able to hear the Holy Spirit's direction for you. To free yourself, take a deep look at your heart and confess any fear, anger, hatred, bitterness or resentment to God through prayer. Ask Him to free you of your burdens, and then ask Him to inhibit Satan from his evil intentions.

Paul talks about this in Ephesians 4:30-32: *"And do not grieve the Holy Spirit of God, with whom you were sealed for the day of redemption. Get rid of all bitterness, rage and anger, brawling and slander, along with every form of malice. Be kind and compassionate to one another, forgiving each other, just as in Christ, God forgave you."*

I found this poem and it seems to fit perfectly with what I am trying to say. Pay particular attention to the Bible verses:

Lord, THEY SAY.

LORD, they say I don't have a child because I don't ask You for one.
CHILD, I say I know you and your needs before you ask me (Matthew 6:8).

LORD, they say I should have a child already because I have been married for a while.
CHILD, I say, "As the heavens are higher than the earth, so are my ways higher than your ways and my thoughts than your thoughts" (Isaiah 55:9).

LORD, they say I have not tried hard enough to have a child.
CHILD, I say it is not human effort which opens a womb. I am the One who grants the gift of children (Psalm 127).

LORD, they say, "Try this—it worked for her; it could work for you."
CHILD, I say, do not fret. Trust me. Be still and know that I am God (Psalm 46).

LORD, they say, "Life is passing you by; many others who are younger than you already have children."
CHILD, I say, "I know the plans I have for you, plans to prosper you and not to harm you, plans to give you hope and a future" (Jeremiah 29:11).

LORD, they say, with sad eyes and looks of pity, "What will you do now?"
CHILD, I say, "My grace is sufficient for you, for my power is made perfect in weakness"
(2 Corinthians 12:9).

Once again, I place my life in His Hands and resolve to live to the fullest, to the praise
and glory of my loving Redeemer.

By Soraya Cina[8]

Chapter Seven—Acknowledging People or Things on God's Throne

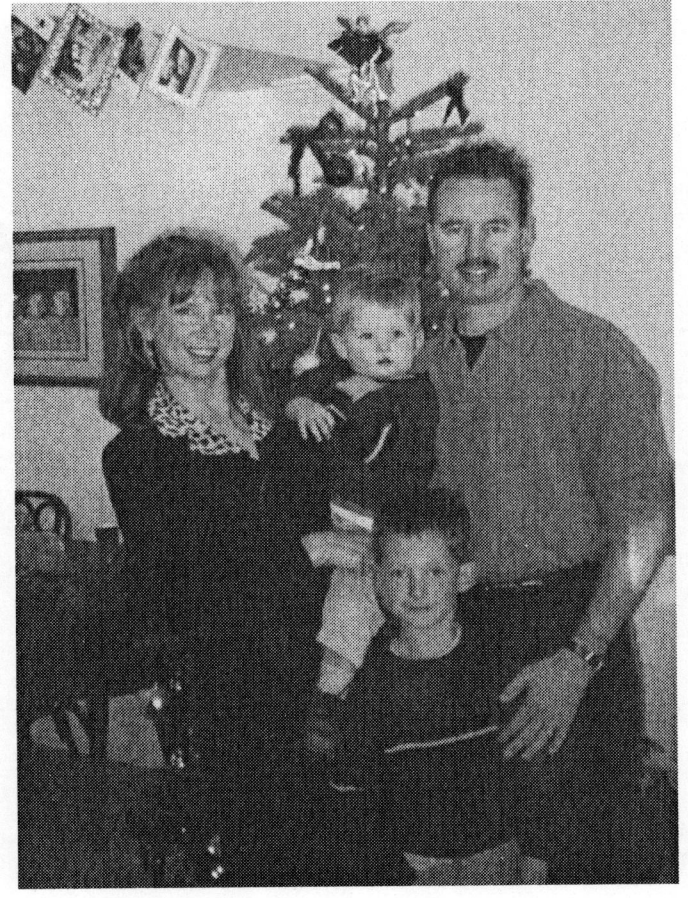

Janet, Parker, Edward and Jake

-Making God Your First Priority
    How to Put God First
-Allowing Your Husband to be Head of the Household
    Drip, Drip, Drip… Taming the Tongue
    Kicking Others or Things Off the Throne

Chapter Seven—Acknowledging People or Things on God's Throne

1. What is the one thing that makes you get out of bed each day? (i.e. what do you live for? – Food? Your hubby? Another day of opportunity to serve God? Your dream of motherhood? Someone in your life? Your aspirations? Nothing?)

_____

_____

_____

2. If you knew that God should be the first priority in your life (the reason you get out of bed), and He isn't, how would you change priorities considering what you listed above? Please explain:

_____

_____

_____

3. Who is the head of your household? (Circle one) a) You b) Your husband c) God d) No one

4. If I told you that God wants you to allow your husband to be the head of your home, what would your first reaction be: a) No way, absolutely not! b) That would be hard for me – I'm a better leader. c) I've tried, but he won't lead! d) I'm working on it, but it takes time. e) He is.

5. If your husband made a decision for your family that you didn't agree with, how would you react? a) I would tell him off. b) I would think about it and then tell him my opinion. c) He's a good decision-maker, so I would acquiesce. d) I would let him have his way and then make him "pay" by holding out on sex. e) Other (please explain:)_____

6. Which areas of infertility are causing you the most stress right now?

_____
_____
_____

7. What other areas of stress do you have in your life? (Work? Marriage? Finances?)

_____
_____
_____

8. Can you change any of the above? Yes or No? If so, how:

_____
_____
_____

9. What seems to trigger your anger, sadness or depression the most? (Your period? Rude comments from others? Seeing pregnant women or babies?)

_____
_____
_____

10. How do you generally "cope" with infertility? (Bubble baths? Talking with friends? Relying on your husband? Reading the Bible?)

_____

_____

_____

Recommended Reading:

Proverbs 21:19, 27:15-16   Matthew 6:24, 31-33
Luke 12:34   John 9:31
1 Corinthians 6:19-20   Ephesians 4:15-16, 5:21-24
Colossians 2:10, 3:18-19   1 Peter 3:1, 8-12
1 John 4:19

Look up this verse and fill in the blanks:

1 Corinthians 11:3: *"Now I want you to realize that the head of every man is Christ, and the head of the woman is _____, and the head of Christ is _____."*

*"**Why** Can't I Have it All?"*
**Answer #6 –A barren womb makes you aware of
people, objects or addictions that "sit on
the throne" of your life – a place reserved for God only.**

Chapter 7—Manoah's Wife's Story

I really wasn't an important person—just a typical Israelite. Unfortunately, what made me different was my inability to bear children. The women in town didn't want to hang out with me, so thankfully the Lord sent me an exceptional husband. Manoah loved me in spite of our disappointment. During my day a woman's identity revolved around her family. Since we had no heirs, Manoah became my life. I couldn't envision living without him!

You can imagine the sheer shock I experienced the day an Angel of the Lord appeared to me! A glorious angel! I felt invisible as a woman and God chose to send an angel to me of all people! His news changed my life forever. He told me that I would have a baby boy! This is what he said, '...the baby is going to be a Nazirite—he will be dedicated to God from the moment of his birth until the day of his death.' [1]

It is purely speculation on my part, but I would guess this woman lead a fairly insignificant life considering that we do not know her first name. However, she was obviously significant in faith and obedience, because the Lord chose her and Manoah to parent Samson.

The Living Bible says: "As a Nazirite, he would take a vow to be set apart for God's service. The angel returned at a later time and informed his mother that her son would begin to rescue the Israelites from the Philistines' oppression. It wasn't until David's day that the Philistine opposition was completely crushed (2 Samuel 8:1). Samson's part in subduing the Philistines was just the beginning, but it was important nonetheless. It was the task God had given Samson to do. This is a great example of faith in following God even if you don't see instant results, because you might be beginning an important job that others will finish."[2]

*"In everything you do, put God first, and he will direct
you and crown your efforts with success."* **Proverbs 3:6 (NLT)**

Making God Your First Priority

Unfortunately, it is easy to give God our leftovers: our leftover time, leftover love, and leftover devotion. As women, we are pulled in so many directions all day long. We need to give God time and our husband attention; some of you have children tugging on you, there's laundry to do, food to cook, demanding bosses, friends calling... it's never ending. You must take the time to think about what is important to you and then make your priority list. What did you list as important to you on question one? Where was God on that list? How did you answer number two? Luke 12:34 (NLT) says, "Wherever your treasure is, there your heart and thoughts will be."

Where do you put your time, money and energy? I was guilty of putting God aside and focusing strictly on getting pregnant. Are you guilty of the same? Are you fooling yourself into believing you'll have time for God after He answers your prayers? Nothing should be placed above a total commitment to living for Christ.

Have you ever put these things before God: self promotion, self indulgence, success, your husband, your children if you are currently a mother, money, security, recreational entertainment, etc? Unfortunately, I have.

It sounds like Manoah's wife did too. Once again I speculate that Manoah was "everything to his wife" only because her identity seemed to have revolved around being his spouse. I have confessed already that I inadvertently put my husband before God during my own struggle. I depended upon him emotionally and ended up driving him away. I literally could not picture going on with my life without him. He was my rock and in reality, only God is my true "rock."

Why? Because He loved me so much that He sent His "only begotten Son" to earth as a ransom for me (and for you). Because of the sin we were born with (thanks to Adam and Eve), we were separated from God. In all of His glory and purity, He could not look at sinners. By dying on the cross, Jesus Christ "saved" every one of us from the wrath of hell. As He hung on the cross, all of our sins were forgiven (past, present and future). Satan owned us until that freeing moment. Some people choose to remain his. They are fools. But the wise know there is a choice and we can allow God to "own" us when we accept Christ as our Savior.

Now here is the tricky part. Many Christians have been saved from going to hell, but they want the "fire insurance" only, they choose to allow sin to "master" their lives. These people will never experience the fully joyful life God intended for them.

To behold true "oneness" with God, He alone must own you (through salvation), and be your master, meaning He is number One to you and the trials and circumstances you experience only make your relationship with Him stronger and your peace of mind steadfast.

How to Put God First

The best way to describe putting Christ first, or putting Him on the "throne" of your life is by an illustration of Tupperware® Coleman created for her Bible study. This is what she shared:

"In our society it is a sign of weakness when a person has a dependency on something. No one wants to feel or appear to be dependent on anything. The real truth is that God created every human soul with an emptiness and void on purpose so that we will search for its filling.

We must realize dependency was not intended to be evil; it was intended to draw us nearer to God, because God is the only One who can truly fill the void. However, when we stumble onto something that seems to offer even a temporary, false filling, we become dependent on it. Since God is the only One who can truly satisfy us, all other attempts to fill our void will not fit and will eventually fail us. That is, until we fill our void with Christ, who makes us whole."

Coleman said that many Christians become discouraged because they accept Christ as their Savior and they still suffer emptiness and need. She believes the problem is that they receive Christ as their Savior but not as the Lord of their lives. The emptiness they, plus you and I, experience is like a throne in our souls. Whatever we put on the throne is what we are trying to fill our emptiness or void with. Only by placing Christ on the throne of our lives will we completely satisfy our need.

However, when our emptiness finally draws us to Christ for filling, it cannot be accomplished if the proper stacking of our Tupperware® is off. The two go hand in hand. If we want to place Christ on the throne of our lives, then we must begin to follow the One in headship over us.

To understand what she is saying, Coleman gives us an illustration of a wife putting God on her throne. This is a great example of "proper Tupperware® stacking:"

CHAPTER 7—ACKNOWLEDGING PEOPLE OR THINGS ON GOD'S THRONE

CHRIST

HUSBAND

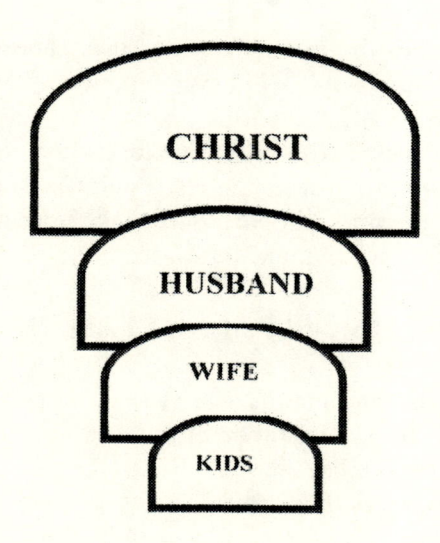

WIFE

KIDS

According to Coleman, by putting God on the throne, this wife:

- Is satisfied because any needs that a man cannot fill, she allows God to fill.
- Lacks for nothing spiritually or emotionally.
- Submits to her husband out of obedience to God.
- Submits not based on her husband's attitude or actions, but based on her relationship with Christ.
- Allows her husband's relationship with Christ to be between him and God, which takes the pressure of performance out of their marriage.

In the above illustration, the top bowl, which personifies Christ, fits over the other three. In other words, Christ is headship over the husband, who is headship over the wife, who is headship over the children. Submission is in the correct order and each is protected and showered with blessings by God. Try taking the Tupperware® bowls and stacking them with any one else on top, and all four bowls will teeter and tumble. If Christ isn't the "top bowl" so to speak, you lose out on His protection and are exposed to God's enemy. God wants to protect you and keep your family from spiritual harm.

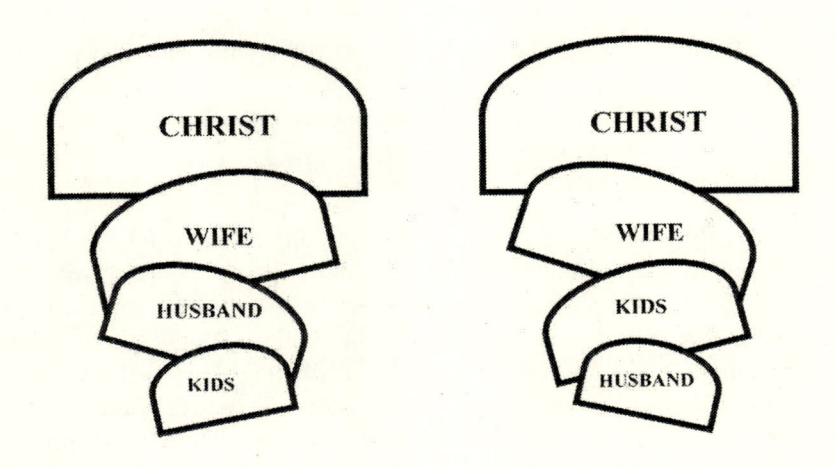

```
    CHRIST              CHRIST
     WIFE                WIFE
   HUSBAND               KIDS
     KIDS              HUSBAND
```

Coleman adds *"A wife cannot say that she has made Christ her Lord when she refuses to be the godly wife God has asked her to be. When the choice is made to place God on the throne of her life, it means her husband must be placed at the head of the table.*

Ladies, it cannot be done any other way and still produce satisfaction in your soul from the 'rivers of living water' quenching your thirst. When you disobey the Lord, your sin separates you from fellowship with Him, so you cannot experience His filling. If you place anything else (or anyone else) besides God on the throne, or stack your Tupperware® in any other way than God's way, the result will be a thirsty soul due to the grieving of the Holy Spirit."

According to Coleman, when a woman places herself on top of the heap, she "wears the pants in the family" and forces her husband out of the leadership role. Because most of us are "control freaks," this is very easy to do, especially if you have a passive husband. The problem is, God didn't design marriage in that order.

She adds, when children "sit on the throne," they rule the roost. This tends to be a very liberal household, where the children are out of control and typically the parents lead separate lives. Likewise, when the desire for children sits on the throne and God is pushed off, once again, your priorities are out of order and you set your household up for attack from the evil one.

Last, when a man is on the throne of your life instead of God, you tend to look to him to fill all of your needs. You tend to cling to him and eventually suffocate him. This kind of headship usually leads to abuse, extramarital affairs on the husband's part, and an unhealthy marriage and spiritual life.

Allowing Your Husband to be Head of the Household

We have talked about putting God first in your life, now let's talk about putting your hubby second as head of the household. Trust me, when my Bible study leader introduced this information to me, I was not a happy camper. I was at a point in my life when I didn't believe I could submit to him, I didn't want to, and I felt he didn't deserve it! Wrong! I learned submission to my husband wasn't about him at all—it's about submitting unto God.

Telling you about submission wasn't my idea. Here's the proof—Ephesians 5:21-23, 25 and 28 tell us to: *"Submit to one another out of reverence for Christ. Wives, submit to your husbands as to the Lord. For the husband is the head of the wife as Christ is the head of the church, his body, of which he is the Savior. Husbands, love your wives, just as Christ loved the church... In this same way, husbands ought to love their wives as their own bodies. He who loves his wife loves himself."*

These verses, as well as Colossians 3:18, say that a wife is to submit to her husband as to the Lord. It doesn't sound like this is a suggestion—it's a command. It is not popular, although that is no reason to discard it.

You might be wondering what submission has to do with infertility, the answer is: everything! You've got to have your house in order. You've got to get yourself to a point where you can surrender. It's interesting to note that all of our lives we submit to people. First, we submit to our parents; second, our teachers; third, authority figures such as police and clergy members; fourth, our superiors at work; fifth, our government leaders, etc. Yet when we are told to submit to our husbands, the hair on the back of our neck stands up!

The first thing I had to learn (after I put God first) was that a man cannot lead his household if he has no followers. I was working out of the home when I learned this, so I was forced to stand up for myself and show aggressiveness at work. It was only natural for me to step in as leader at home and I had to learn and practice following my husband, which in turn, forced him into his rightful leadership position.

The second thing I learned came from Genesis 3:8-9. Adam was the head of the household, so he was responsible for Eve's actions when she ate the apple. Even today, the head of the household, the husband, will be held accountable to God regarding the sins of his family. I don't want that responsibility, do you? That made it easier for me to slide in behind him and let the pressures of the household finances, spiritual direction, etc., fall on my husband's shoulders.

Third, God sends direction for the family through the head of the household—the husband. I've seen it numerous times in my own marriage and in others'. Here are a few ways to make your husband the head of your household and the second in priority in your life:

1. Consult him before making decisions for your family.
2. Have discussions. If you disagree with him after making a family decision, state your opinion and then go with his decision. (Remember, he will ultimately be held accountable.)
3. If he does make the wrong decision, bite your tongue and don't tell him "I told you so!" The more decisions he makes, the better he'll get at making good ones.
4. Try not to be contrite, whining or nagging.
5. If you are better at paying bills and keeping the finances in order, ask him to make the decisions and then you follow through with payments and reconciliation.
6. Do not complain about him to your friends, and especially don't put him down or make fun of him in public.
7. If he acts like a jerk, bite your tongue and force yourself to refrain from giving him an earful.
8. Listen to his complaints and take appropriate actions if necessary.
9. If you have children, talk together before making disciplinary decisions on your own.
10. Make your master bedroom a place where you two can be romantic—don't leave piles of clothing all over the floor or stacks of paper lying around. If you have children, don't place their pictures on the walls of your bedroom. It's difficult for most of us to feel or act sexy when we're staring at our children's faces. Decorate your "love pit" in a manner pleasing to both of you. Another example includes your choice of décor. I once decorated our master bedroom with flowered wallpaper, flowered sheets, and other girly touches. My husband didn't feel it was his room too, so when I redecorated, I asked what his wishes were first and compromised.

CHAPTER 7—ACKNOWLEDGING PEOPLE OR THINGS ON GOD'S THRONE

11. Make him a part of this ordeal without forcing doctors appointments, testing and sex on demand upon him. Let him have a voice in the matter.
12. Ask him how he feels about the whole infertility process and see where he stands. Is he grieving too? If he has learned he is sterile, ask what his wishes are instead of demanding other options. I would hate for you to find out he was contemplating divorce or even suicide after it's too late.

Look back at Claudia's testimony in Chapter 4. It is an excellent example of a woman allowing God to send His will for the family through her husband. When I was teaching on this subject at my infertility Bible study, another great example unfolded before our eyes.

One of the ladies in the group, Janet, got a call from a lawyer about a little girl whose mother could not keep her. Janet and her husband went and met the mother and Janet played with the baby girl and held her tight in her arms. She had a son at home and dearly wanted a baby girl to join him. She and her husband left the woman's home and Janet asked her husband what he thought. He said it didn't feel right to him. She told our group later that she wanted that baby girl so badly that she had to bite her tongue and respect her husband's headship. We all respected her so much and we got to witness the blessings that came to her family after that. It was the right decision.

Janet submitted and God honored her. You see we each have an audience of ONE. He is the only One you and I should try to please. Submission is done out of reverence to God, not because your husband deserves it (although he might). If you do it for your husband, it will become conditional submission. If you submit out of obedience to God, it will produce eternal blessings.

Think of a bicycle. The hub is the core onto which the spokes support the tire. The center, or the hub, gives the tire balance, support and strength. Take a deep look at your life and decide what your "hub" is. If God is the center of your life, you will be balanced and pedaling steady and strong through this difficult season in your life.

The Road of Life

At first, I saw God as my observer, my judge
keeping track of the things I did wrong, so as to know
whether I merited heaven or hell when I die. He was out
there sort of like a president. I recognized His
picture when I saw it, but I really didn't know him.

But later on when I met Christ it seemed as
though life were like a bike ride, but it was a tandem
bike, and I noticed that Christ was in the back helping me pedal.

I don't know just when it was that he suggested
we change places, but life has not been the same since.
When I had control, I knew the way. It was
rather boring, but predictable… It was the shortest
distance between two points.

But when He took the lead, He knew delightful
long cuts, up mountains, and through rocky places at
breakneck speeds, it was all I could do to hang on!
Even though it looked like madness He said, "Pedal!"
I was worried and was anxious and asked
"Where are you taking me?" He laughed and didn't
answer, and I started to learn to trust.

I forgot my boring life and entered into the
adventure. And when I'd say, "I'm scared," He'd lean
back and touch my hand.

He took me to people with gifts that I needed,
gifts of healing, acceptance and joy. They gave me gifts
to take on my journey, my Lord's and mine.

And we were off again. He said, "Give the gifts
away; they're extra baggage, too much weight." So I
did, to the people we met, and I found that in giving I
received, and still our burden was light.

CHAPTER 7—ACKNOWLEDGING PEOPLE OR THINGS ON GOD'S THRONE

I did not trust him at first in control of my
life. I thought He'd wreck it; but he knows bike
secrets, knows how to make it bend to take sharp
corners, knows how to jump to clear high rocks, knows
how to fly to shorten scary passages.

And I am learning to shut up and pedal in the
strangest places, and I'm beginning to enjoy the view
and the cool breeze on my face with my delightful
constant companion, Jesus Christ.

And when I'm sure I just can't do anymore,
He just smiles and says.... "Pedal."

Author unknown

Drip, Drip, Drip...Taming the Tongue

A few weeks ago I found myself in an unpleasant situation. It sounded like this: You mean you want me to iron your shirts? I already have enough on my plate! I'm trying to keep the house clean, keep all of us fed right, feed the dogs, pay the bills, deal with the kids, do the laundry... and there was my poor husband looking at me as if I was some kind of lunatic. I was a lunatic— a dripping one!
Look at these Proverbs verses from *The Living Bible* translation:

27:15-16—*"A constant dripping on a rainy day and a cranky woman are much alike! You can no more stop her complaints than you can stop the wind or hold onto anything with oil-slick hands."*
19:13—*"A rebellious son is a calamity to his father, and a nagging wife annoys like constant dripping."*
21:9—*"It is better to live in the corner of the attic than with a crabby woman in a lovely home."*
21:19—*"Better to live in the desert than with a quarrelsome, complaining woman."*
25:24—*"It is better to live in the corner of an attic than in a beautiful home with a cranky, quarrelsome woman."*

Have you ever been with a girlfriend and heard her go on and on about her husband, or been out in public and she's telling people confidential and unflattering things about him? Don't you just want to slap her and say, Wake up you idiot? You've got a great man and you're going to drive him away! I have been there. And guess what? I've been on the other end too. I still catch myself to this day complaining about my hubby and referring to him in less than respectful ways. I don't want to be foolish like that. It's unflattering and it ruins my Christian witness.

The action we women must learn to take every minute of every day is controlling our tongues. It's so hard to do. Most of us want "the last word," we can be vicious with a single sentence, and most of us build ourselves up, by tearing others down.

You might be wondering why I'm bringing this up; it is because in your vulnerable state, Lucifer will use the wickedness of your tongue against you, your husband, your friends and your family. I want to teach you to be alert and aware.

The Living Bible has this to say about the "Four Tongues:" *"What we say probably affects more people than any other action we take. It is not surprising, then, to find that Proverbs gives special attention to words and how they are used. Four common speech patterns are described in Proverbs. The first two should be copied, while the last two should be avoided:"*

1. The Controlled Tongue—Those with this speech pattern think before speaking, know when silence is best, and give wise advice. Proverbs—10:14, 19; 11:12,13; 12:16; 13:3; 15:1, 4, 28; 16:23; 17:14, 27, 28; 18:4; 21:23; 24:26; 26:17.

2. The Caring Tongue—Those with this speech pattern speak truthfully while seeking to encourage. Proverbs – 10:32; 12:18, 25; 15:23, 26; 16:24; 25:15; 27:9.

3. The Conniving Tongue—Those with this speech pattern are filled with wrong motives, gossip, slander and they twist the truth. Proverbs—6:12-14; 8:13; 16:28; 18:8; 25:18; 26:4, 5, 20-28.

4. The Careless Tongue—Those with this speech pattern are filled with lies, curses and quick-tempered words – which can lead to rebellion and destruction. Proverbs—10:18, 32; 11:9; 12:16,18; 15:4; 17:9, 14, 19; 18:21; 20:19; 25:23.[3]

Peter said, *"If you want a happy, good life, keep control of your tongue, and guard your lips from telling lies,"* (1 Peter 3:10 NLT). Why is it so hard for women to do this? The answer is: because of the curse on Eve. Look at this verse:

"...Your desire will be for your husband, and he will rule over you," (Genesis 3:16b). The word "desire" in this verse refers to his position. Our desire to control is purely natural and it's a curse we have to wrestle with—and beat down in this case.

My Bible says: *"The book of Proverbs begins with the command to trust and reverence the Lord (1:7) and ends with a picture of a woman who fulfills this command. Her qualities are mentioned throughout the book: hard work, fear of God, respect for spouse, foresight, encouragement, care for others, concern for the poor, wisdom in handling money. These qualities, when coupled with fear of God [reverence], lead to enjoyment, success, honor, and worth. Proverbs is very practical for our day because it shows us how to become wise, make good decisions, and live according to God's ideal."*[4]

What we are dealing with here is our sinful nature, which is referred to as "our flesh." It wants to be number one by doing what is desirable and pleasurable, yet God wants and needs to be first in your life. Therefore, He tells us in His Word what is off limits and what is pleasing to Him.

Choosing the latter will keep you out of trouble!

Kicking Others or Things Off the Throne

If and when you realize that something, someone, or your "flesh" (your sinful nature), is number one in your life instead of God, you need to kick them off the "throne" and give God His rightful place. The first thing to do is confess this error to God and ask for forgiveness. Second, ask Him to help you. His Holy Spirit will direct you and help you in the process.

Let's say that an addiction controls you. For example, a woman who can't get through a day of her life without pain killers has let them control her. God gave us self control for a reason. This person, if she was really serious, would need to seek professional help so that she was once again able to live for God instead of numbing herself to "get through the day."

I have often witnessed women with past hurts such as incest, child molestation and rape who are paralyzed with unforgiveness. This is understandable, yet they usually don't realize it and rarely admit it that unforgiveness rules them. Unforgiveness and the blazing anger and bitterness that accompany it control their lives. These women will never experience true peace in their lives until they come to grips with the overwhelming bondage, confess it, and forgive their offenders once and for all. I'm not saying this would be easy, however, it is very necessary.

A woman who has the dream of motherhood as her sole focus is another example. She can be like a horse with blinders on. My testimony is the perfect example. I put my marriage aside during the chase, I was a "fake" around my friends, my focus was on what I didn't have, and God had to really shake me up to get my attention. No wonder it was a long road before I realized my error.

It seems that God had to get Dixie's attention too: *"It took me years to realize that my biggest struggle with infertility was with self-pity. It robbed God of his rightful place on the throne of my heart and replaced Him with Self. Self-pity says to God that He is blind to our suffering and is unwilling to do what is in our best interest. Self-pity robs us of the healing and the joy that takes place when we put all our trust in Him. No wonder self-pity is a sin."*[5]

Think seriously about your life. Write down your habits, your goals, your motives for motherhood, and your priorities. Study the list and ask God if there is unconfessed sin in your life. If there is, trust me, in a couple days or so, He will reveal it to you. Stop right then and confess it immediately. Afterward, you will be "one" with God again, and he will be able to answer you when you ask what areas of your life are out of control or in the wrong order.

Finally, Coleman adds *"Misalignment of your proper rank and order (your Tupperware®), equals areas of vulnerability to the enemy."* On the other hand, *"When you are in proper rank and order, the enemy must go through Christ to get to you. You are completely protected under Christ."*

> **"Now I want you to realize that the head of every man is Christ, and the head of the woman is man, and the head of Christ is God."**
> **1 Corinthians 11:3**

Chapter Eight–Humbling Yourself Unto the Lord

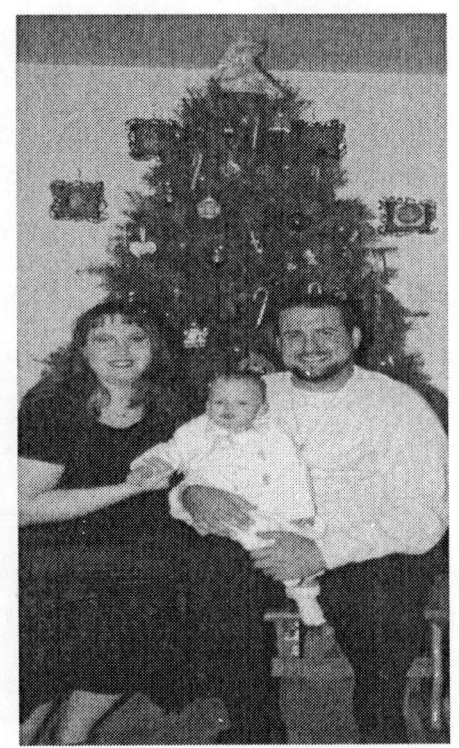

Charlene, Ernie, Kayla

-Being Humble When You Feel Broken
    How to Overcome Anger, Jealousy and Unforgiveness
    How to Keep Your Friends During this Season
    How to Tell Your Infertile Friends You Are Pregnant
    Practical Advice for Barren Women
    Practical Advice for Couples Struggling with Infertility
-Being Prepared for Insensitive Remarks and Suggestions
-Attending Child-Centered Occasions
    Handling Child-Centered Holidays
    Dealing with Christmas

Chapter Eight–Humbling Yourself Unto the Lord

1. Do you try to "work" your way to heaven by doing good deeds or by being a "good girl?" Yes or No?

2. Have you accepted Christ and given Him your life? Yes or No?

3. Define "humility" in your own terms (don't use a dictionary):

_____

_____

_____

4. Are you jealous of someone right now? Please list their name(s):

_____

_____

_____

5. Name the people you are or have been angry with:

_____

_____

_____

6. Do you feel desperate for a child? Yes or No? Do you feel desperate for God? Yes or No?

7. How do you generally handle unsolicited, insensitive remarks and suggestions?

_____

_____

_____

8. What holidays or occasions are the most difficult for you? Name them please:

_____

_____

_____

9. What could you do to make them easier to handle (other than getting pregnant):

_____

_____

_____

Recommended Reading:

Psalm 34, 84:11	Proverbs 14:10, 19:11, 15:33, 27:4
Isaiah 40:29	Matthew 5:10
Luke 14:11	Ephesians 4:17-32
Titus 3:2	Hebrews 12:15
James 3:2-10, 14-16, 4:1-12	1 Peter 3:9

CHAPTER 8—HUMBLING YOURSELF UNTO THE LORD

Look up these verses and fill in the blanks:

Psalm 34:18-19 (NLT): *"The Lord is close to those whose hearts are breaking; he rescues those who are _____ sorry for their sins. The good man does not escape all troubles – he has them too. But the Lord helps him in each and every one."*

Ephesians 4:31-32: *"Get rid of all _____, rage and anger, brawling and slander, along with every form of malice. Be kind and compassionate to one another, forgiving each other, just as in Christ God forgave you."*

Colossians 3:13: *"Bear with each other and _____ whatever grievances you may have against one another. Forgive as the Lord _____ you."*

"Why *do I Hurt so Bad?"*
Answer #7 – A barren womb forces you to humble yourself unto the Lord by eliminating unforgiveness, jealousy and anger.

Chapter 8–Rachel's Story

My husband, Jacob, worked for my father for seven years so he could marry me and then on our wedding night my father tricked us. When Jacob agreed to work off my dowry, my father deceived him by choosing not to divulge that the oldest daughter must be married first. Thus, on the night of our honeymoon, my father took my elder sister, Leah, to Jacob while it was dark and he didn't realize that he was sleeping with the wrong sister until morning.

Jake was a good and honorable man, so he agreed to work for my father for another seven years so that he could marry me too. What got me through those days was the knowledge that Jacob loved me. In fact, everyone knew he loved me more then Leah. The only problem was she had baby after baby for him and I remained barren. It just wasn't right. I was so hurt I just wanted to die. I had to catch up with Leah, so I decided to take matters into my own hands. I gave my servant girl, Bilhah, to Jacob to sleep with and she bore him two sons—Dan and Naphtali.

My arms ached to hold my own baby and smell his precious scent. I longed to experience life within me and I agonized as I watched my sister, Leah, pregnant seven times. I looked at my own niece and nephews with hostility and resentment in my heart. I could not be happy for my sister. Her baby showers were constant reminders of my inadequacy. Zilpah (Leah's servant girl) bore two more sons. Bilhah birthed two sons as well and my womb remained empty. I could not rebuke jealousy, envy or resentment. My life seemed worthless.

The waiting seemed endless and I wondered if I would ever be a "normal wife" to Jake. My anger was so intense. I was angry at my body for betraying me. I was angry at my family for having reunions brimming with children who were not mine. I was angry at Jacob for making babies with Leah. And, for awhile, I was angry at the Lord for allowing me to hurt so badly.

Finally, Jehovah remembered me and opened my womb so that I could give birth to my sons: Joseph and Benjamin. My prayers had finally been answered and I praised the Lord![1]

The biography of Rachel in *The Living Bible* points out interesting characteristics of her life: *"Jacob's love for Rachel was both patient and practical. Jacob had the patience to wait seven years for her, but he kept busy in the meantime. His commitment to Rachel kindled a strong loyalty within her. In fact, her loyalty to Jacob got out of hand and became self-destructive. She was frustrated by her barrenness and desperate to compete with her sister for Jacob's affection. She was trying to gain from Jacob what he had already given: devoted love.*

Rachel's attempts to earn the unearnable are a picture of a much greater error we can make. Like her, we find ourselves trying somehow to earn love—God's love. But apart from his Word, we end up with one of two false ideas: Either we think we've been good enough to deserve his love, or we recognize we aren't able to earn his love and assume that it cannot be ours.

If the Bible makes no other point, it shouts this one: God loves us! His love has no beginning and is incredibly patient. All we need to do is respond, not try to earn what is freely offered. God has said in many ways, 'I love you. I have demonstrated that love to you by all I've done for you. I have even sacrificed my Son, Jesus, to pay the price for what is unacceptable about you (your sin). Now, live because of my love. Respond to me; love me with your whole being; give yourself to me in thanks, not as payment. Live life fully, in the freedom of knowing you are loved.'"[2]

"Leaving Bethel, he [Jacob] and his household traveled on toward Ephrath (Bethlehem). But Rachel's pains of childbirth began while they were still a long way away. After a very hard delivery, the midwife finally exclaimed, 'Wonderful—another boy!' And with Rachel's last breath (for she died) she named him 'Ben-oni' (Son of my sorrow'); but his father called him 'Benjamin' ('Son of my right hand')."
Genesis 35:16-18 (NLT).

Being Humble When You Feel Broken

Rachel allowed jealousy of her sister and desperation for her husband to rule her life. We must learn a lesson from her as we humble ourselves and become desperate for God, instead of a baby, more children, our husband or things of this world.

I'm confident you know what humility is, therefore I'll tell you what it is not. Humility is not prideful, quarrelsome, jealous, unforgiving, or uncontrolled. Rachel exemplified all of these characteristics and look where it got her—she died giving birth to her second son whom she named Ben-oni (son of my sorrow). On the other hand, her sister, Leah, the unloved wife of Jacob realized that she could never win her husband's love. She turned her focus from what she didn't have to what she had—God's love. When naming her maidservant's second son, Leah announced "*How happy I am*" and it was her lineage that led to the birth of Christ.

Leah learned that becoming desperate for God involved drawing near to Him. Read James 4:1-10 (NLT). Verses three and four really got my attention: James said in verse three that sometimes we don't get what we want because our aim is wrong—we want something for selfish pleasure. What were your motives for motherhood as discussed in Chapter 2? I would be willing to bet the majority of you never stopped to think about it. I would also wager that most of you have great motives. If you don't, take a deep look within yourself.

Additionally verse four reads: "*You are like an unfaithful wife who loves her husband's enemies. Don't you realize that making friends with God's enemies – the evil pleasures of this world—makes you an enemy of God? I say it again, that if your aim is to enjoy the evil pleasures of the unsaved world, you cannot also be a friend of God.*" From our vantage point, I believe this would refer to calling yourself a good person or even a Christian and then allowing yourself to be consumed with infertility's natural responses: pride, quarreling, jealousy, an unforgiving spirt, and uncontrolled behavior (such as outbursts, anger, slander, etc.).

The Living Bible tells us that James gives five suggestions on how to practice humility and draw closer to God:

Give yourself humbly to God—Realize that you need his forgiveness, and be willing to follow Him even when times are tough or when you feel distant from Him.

Resist the devil—Don't allow him to entice and tempt you. Stay away from people, things or areas that tempt you.

Wash your hands (that is lead a pure life) and let your hearts be filled with God—Be cleansed from sin, replacing it with God's purity.

Let there be tears, sorrow, and sincere grief for your sins— Don't be afraid to express deep, heartfelt sorrow for sin.

Realize your worthlessness—Humble yourself before God and he will lift you up (1 Peter 5:6).[3]

When you are humble before the Lord, He can use you. If you are desperate for anything else, you've given the devil a foothold and he'll use *and abuse you*. Desperation is a strong feeling, like an ache in the pit of your stomach. It's easy to make snap judgments and even poorly thought out decisions when you are in this state.

For instance, I remember sitting in an adoption agency agreeing to terms a birth mother wanted for her child that I was completely uncomfortable with and that I had disagreed to on earlier occasions. There was an uneasiness in the pit of my stomach and I walked away from that appointment feeling ashamed of myself for demonstrating such a lack of integrity. Of course, that adoption did not take place because God knew I was playing the desperate game. To feel desperate for God, the feelings are the same—they're just in the right context.

Desperation for God is basically understanding that He alone will complete you. Through humility He will embrace you, and as you pray to Him, you will begin to ache for a deepened relationship with Him. You know you're there when you find yourself depending on Him for everything aspect of your life.

CHAPTER 8—HUMBLING YOURSELF UNTO THE LORD

How to Overcome Anger, Jealousy and Unforgiveness

I'm sure you are hurt, maybe even crushed by the devastation of infertility or pregnancy loss. You are more than likely experiencing feelings of anger, jealousy and unforgiveness with the people in your world. You might even feel uncomfortable admitting anger – that in doing do so, God will surely strike you with lightning. Try not to be so hard on yourself. What you are experiencing is new and it's undeniably "larger than life" I'm sure.

In the book, *What to Expect When You're Experiencing Infertility,*[4] the authors, Debby Peoples and Harriette Rovner Ferguson, C.S.W., wrote great advice I want to pass on to you: *"Getting past your disappointmet and anger toward God in order to get closer to Him is not easy... the best way to do this is to accept the fact that you are angry. This can be a difficult task for those who grew up believing that such anger was blasphemous and could cause God in His ire to retaliate in some way. Letting God know how angry and upset you are is an acceptable, understandable part of the letting-go process that must take place in order for you to make peace with your spirituality."*

The letter you are about to read might seem disturbing, but I feel it's a great example of what the authors just said:

Dear God, As you most certainly know by now, I don't have any faith whatsoever in you. I don't even like you. I think you've done a lousy job of supervising the frail planet on which I live. Under normal circumstances, you'd be fired. You must have terrific tenure.

Nonetheless, I couldn't find anybody else old enough and big enough to talk to. I've noticed a lot of other humans whispering to you, mumbling their thanks, quietly requesting everything from profit-sharing to eternal salvation. I'm not asking for anything. I just want to let you know that I'm angry. Filled with rage that's got twenty thousand years of savage mating behind it. And I want to explode it at your heaven.

I cannot have children. Like Abraham's wife, Sarah. Remember her? A barren womb, empty arms. Of all the plagues and curses and disasters you have sent to earth, this is the most wicked. It is incomprehensible.

Nothing you schemed was quite as treacherous as the human heart. You connected it to everything. Every sight and every gesture, every cell in every tissue in every organ in every body registers somewhere in the heart. To touch a new baby, to contemplate eternity, to ovulate, to bury a grandmother, to love a man— these, and a thousand other events coagulate, and somewhere in the thick purple muscle of the heart, form a longing: to have children.

It is not an irrational desire. It is, in fact, the natural order of things. It is unnatural only inside a woman who is barren. Then this longing, this sweet harmless longing, turns on itself, clogs the opening to the heart, spreads over the entire surface of the heart, hardening many of the tender spots, breaking it in places, and finally, in desperation, exploding. All that is left is a great gaping hole that will never be filled. You ask more than is reasonable. Amen."

Now that is honesty. This woman isn't telling God anything He doesn't already know about her feelings, yet she's letting her fury out. She's angry enough to spout words she probably doesn't even mean, yet she's choosing a healthy facet rather than ignoring her inner feelings.

Anger—The Bible doesn't tell us we shouldn't feel angry (Jesus was even angered while on this earth—see John 2:15), but it is important to handle your anger properly. For example, if you let it explode, you risk destroying relationships (think of Rachel and Leah). If you leave it bottled up inside, it can cause you to become bitter and it will destroy you from within. That's why harsh words like those in the letter above can be healthy.

I want you to make a list. Write in the names of anyone whom you have been rude to, or whom you are angry with, or whom you refuse to forgive. Don't read on until you make it your sincere intention to take this list, as well as the names you listed on questions four and five, and: a) forgive them, b) ask for their forgiveness, and c) let go of the anger and/or bitterness and move on:

Doctor _____	Nurse _____
Technician _____	Friend _____
Neighbor _____	Relative _____
Husband _____	Yourself _____
God _____	Others _____

"We often have the wrong idea about anger. We think 'truly spiritual people feel only positive emotions,' but it's not immature to feel angry; it's immature to stay angry," said Sandy Glahn, co-author of *When Empty Arms Become a Heavy Burden*.[5]

Jealousy—I can understand Rachel's envy of Leah's children, however, her jealousy was out of place. Jacob loved her, and in her efforts to compete in the child-bearing race, she sinned by giving him her maidservant. Be wise and don't let jealousy lead you into sin. Paul tells us in Romans 13:12-14 not to underestimate jealousy. He lists it along with obvious sins such as drunkenness, fighting and adultery.

Read how Debbie was released from her feelings of jealousy: *"My husband and I have been experiencing secondary infertility for the last four years. When we first realized that infertility was a part of our lives, my eyes could only see all of the women around me who were becoming pregnant and multiplying their families. My heart ached every time another friend came to me, sharing the news of her pregnancy.*

Try as I might to not be jealous or hurt, those were the first feelings I identified with when the news came. It wasn't until my prayer partner told me she was pregnant that my feelings hit a wall; and the way that I dealt with them was changed forever. My prayer partner, to whom I had grown particularly close, had one child and she and her husband were not going to have any more, so I felt she was 'on my side.'

God asked me a simple question, 'What does your friend's pregnancy have to do with how I feel about you?' 'What?' I asked God. 'What do you mean?' And God showed me how, in my error of comparing my life to others—even biblical others, I was erasing a truth so crucial to my walk with God.

I knew that God was saying to me, 'I love you, apart from anyone else. You are special, apart from anyone else. I have a plan for you, apart from anyone else. When you look at others and think your life is so unfair, remember that I love you, I love you, I love you! Your value to me has nothing to do with anyone else, not even with anything that you are or that you can do. It has only to do with ME!'

Wow! This was so huge and freeing for me! My value to God has nothing to do with my getting pregnant. My value to God has nothing to do with how I compare my life to others. I was free from the trap of comparison... the trap that always made me jealous and the trap that inevitably made me feel like an ungrateful wretch. For the first time, I began to see the lie that I believed about my worth to God. Isn't that exactly what the enemy wanted me to believe?"[6]

I have two additional pieces of advice: First, look at the names you listed on question nunber four and make every effort to get past your jealousy toward them. Satan will use envy to snare you, once successful, he'll usually introduce guilt to finally trap you. Talk to the Lord about when you feel this kind of resentment; you might even consider talking to someone about your feelings or even sharing your envy with the person(s) involved.

Second, the next time you walk past a pregnant lady or a woman with a baby, ask yourself these questions: *I wonder if she had trouble getting pregnant? I wonder if she walked in my shoes and her prayers were answered? I wonder if her baby was adopted?* I've been glared at so many times because I had a newborn in my stroller and displayed no signs of weight gain. Remember, things aren't always what they seem.

Unforgiveness—We all experience the inconsiderate, mean, things people say to us or suggest, right? For instance, on two different occasions a man found out I couldn't conceive and had the audacity to say, *"Hey baby, if your old man isn't getting the job done, let me show you how to do it."* Yes, that really happened!

Usually women's comments sting me more than men's, but not in this case. Instead of slapping this man in the face or kicking him in the groin, I usually said, *"No thanks, it will all work out in God's timing,"* and quickly walked away. This usually ruined his fun and made him think twice about his barbaric suggestions.

It's hard to look at people in the same way after they've offended you. I had to remind myself that these people were just ignorant. They didn't know what they were talking about, so they used joking as a way to alleviate the uneasiness they might have been feeling. Instead of holding a grudge in situations like this, I had to remind myself that God loves them as much as He loves me.

Look at this warning regarding unforgiveness and the enemy's schemes in 2 Corinthians 2:9-11: *"The reason I wrote you was to see if you would stand the test and be obedient in everything. If you forgive anyone, I also frogive him. And what I have forgiven – if there was anything to forgive – I have forgiven in the sight of Christ for your sake, in order that Satan might not outwit us. For we are not unaware of his schemes."*

God may be testing you to refine you like silver (Psalm 66:10),[7] and it is important that you be strong and courageous. *"Set your mind on things above, not on earthly things,"* (Colossians 3:2) and remind yourself that you are so loved. Why else would God take the time to purify you and make you spotless and refined?[8]

Last, ask God to help you look at the lists of names you made and not only forgive each person, but see them as He sees them—blameless!

CHAPTER 8—HUMBLING YOURSELF UNTO THE LORD

How to Keep Your Friends During This Season

Joy Englesman wrote an aritcle titled, "Lonely or Loved – Maintaining Friendships Through the Infertility Journey." Because I feel it is important to avoid loneliness, and because I feel you should allow others to bear your burdens, I want to share her ideas with you. Joy lost her third child to miscarriage. Needless to say, she and her husband, Bob, were heartbroken. *"We were separated from our family by thousands of miles and from our friends by their silence, we felt as if we were the last two people on the face of the earth."*

Englesman said infertility tests all areas of life: physical, emotional, financial, and spiritual. It also has the dangerous power to totally devastate a couple's social life. Often, friendships are defined by what we have in common. This is a most dangerous definition for the infertile couple.

She adds, *"First, no one wants to belong to such a 'club,' so the 'membership' is reluctant, reticent, resistant—not exactly the kind of people to support you in need. Second, sooner or later, members of the club will graduate—either through pregnancy or adoption—leaving the remaining members feeling more isolated. A circle of friendship based exclusively on common experiences with infertility may serve well as a temporary support group, but it usually won't last the test of time."*

So how can we redefine our friendships so they endure? What can we do to help our friends who want to love us, but are hesitant to do so because of the depth and intensity of our pain? She says, ***"to get a friend, you must be a friend.***

My husband and I realized early on that if we wanted to keep our friends we would have to be honest with them about our pain, our hopes, and our hurts. We wished they would have known what to say or do without telling them, but we learned that they needed us to teach them about infertility and grief.

Our best friends are the people who trust us by being real with us. They don't walk on eggshells around us. They dare to laugh with us, cry with us, ask for our prayers for them, and promise the same for us. They invite us to share their lives, hold their babies, play with their children, and they understand when we can't.

These are the friends I called after my last miscarriage, when we heard from no one after five days. They listened when I told them that I was feeling abandoned, and they were sorry that they hadn't called and responded with love and compassion. Together we learned more about forgiveness and how deeply honest we would have to be if we were going to remain friends. We'll continue to risk stepping on each other's toes just to have the chance to join in the dance."

Englesman concludes by saying, "*Our friends have walked with us through the highs and lows of infertility, and through it all we have sensed God's presence in their sincere efforts to remain faithful. We pray that He has used us to build His earthly family, as we learn to release our grip on our pain and share it with those He has called to be our friends. May you find the friends you need to carry you, too."*[9]

How to Tell Your Infertile Friends You Are Pregnant

"*Soldiers who enter combat together often speak of a bond that forms between them because of what they have faced together. In many ways there is a similar bond between those who face the struggle of infertility,*" said Sylvia Van Regenmorter who wrote an article I want to share with you titled "I'm Pregnant, How Do I Tell My Infertile Friends?"

Van Regenmorter recalls her two closest friends: Bev and Pam, both "*fellow travelers along the road of infertility.*" She says that for three years they worked together, cried together, and prayed together.

"*Then, suddenly, long after we had given up on medical intervention, John and I became pregnant. I was elated but I was also troubled. I wondered: How would I tell my best friends? What would their reaction be? Would it hurt our friendship? Should I keep them informed and involved in my pregnancy?*" she wondered.

Since then Van Regenmorter has come up with the following advice. "*I am not suggesting that there is a 'right way' or a 'wrong way' to deal with friends after you become pregnant,*" she said, "*I do hope, however, that the following will give you some help to face this delicate challenge:*"

• Be prepared for some mixed emotions. I was excited to be pregnant after so many years, yet my heart hurt for my friends who were still in pain. I thought there was something wrong with me that I could not fully enjoy my pregnancy. Since that time I have learned that my feelings were normal. The sad fact is that years of infertility rob many couples of the full joy of pregnancy because they are sensitive to others who continue to wait with empty arms.

- Make sure your friends hear the news from you directly and not from a mutual acquaintance or through the 'grapevine.' Nothing is more hurtful than to hear about a friend's pregnancy from someone else.

"When I became pregnant, one of the first things I did was talk to Bev and Pam, face to face, to share the news with them. We laughed together and we cried. It was difficult but I know they were extremely grateful that they were among the first to know. As Bev said, 'This gives me time to prepare before the whole world knows.' Honesty is always the best policy. If you do not quite know what to say to your friend, tell her that. If you are not sure how involved she wants to be in your pregnancy, ask her what involvement she would like to have."

- Be aware that, after you become pregnant, maintaining a close relationship with an infertile friend is a challenge! I am not suggesting that you cannot remain close friends, but it will take work and energy from both sides. After you become pregnant, your focus changes to ultrasounds, fixing up the baby's room, and morning sickness. Your friend may still be riding the (seemingly) never-ending roller coaster of hope and disappointment. Either of you must be careful and intentional about your friendship or it will be easy to drift apart.

"Even though I have now moved to a city far away from my friends and our lives have gone in different directions, my friendships with Bev and Pam have been and continue to be a treasure."[10]

Practical Advice for Barren Women

It is imperative that you learn to cope with this issue. I remember being so freaked out that I feared my husband would commit me to an insane asylum. When you look at the stresses of everyday life and then factor in the emotional stress of infertility, and the "oh so fun" tests we get to go through, plus the expense of those tests, then your period arriving the day of your best friend's baby shower, it's just too much for anyone to handle.

Trusting that *"He [God] gives power to the tired and worn out, and strength to the weak"* (Isaiah 40:29 NLT), helped me, however, I believe God wants us to do our part too. The ladies who have provided testimonials for this book advise the following coping mechanisms:

1. Go for long walks
2. Take weekend trips

3. Do things that make you happy (manicures, pedicures, massages, picnics)
4. Consider getting a pet
5. Take long bubble baths
6. Consider taking classes
7. Join a care group at your church or a support group
8. Exercise
9. Try to eliminate stressful areas in your life
10. Refocus on your job or career.
11. Take the focus off your menstrual cycle, hormone levels and tests and refocus on getting your life back. One way to do this is to take 20 minutes a day to sit quietly and relax. Take time to breathe and be mindful of the present instead of what's coming up or what hasn't happened.
12. Pamper your husband with his favorite meals and favorite past times. Make your marriage a priority and remind yourself to cherish your husband.
13. Take time to read. Two recommended books were: *Healthy Mind Healthy Woman* by Dr. Alice Domar and *Light in My Darkest Night* by Catherine Marshall.
14. If you have a child, throw a surprise party or sleepover just for the fun of it. Remember that sometimes while the months and years pass and you are going through test after test and treatment after treatment, the focus is so great on becoming pregnant again that you suddenly realize time has passed and you missed special moments with the child(ren) you have.
15. Take up new hobbies (ceramics, bowling, scrap booking, camping, gardening)
16. When you plan to go shopping or attend gatherings including children, prepare your mind in advance. Also be prepared for insensitive questions and remarks by following the advice later in this chapter.
17. When speaking with your husband about your situation, apply the 20-minute rule described later in this chapter.
18. Journal your thoughts, emotions, disappointments and blessings
19. Keep praying with listening ears and reading your Bible and meditating on key verses

The best advice I can give is getting to the point when you have surrendered your life to God and are experiencing peace. It's a place where you can finally give God the navigational duties in your life. When you're at peace with yourself, your marriage and your life; you're less tense, less confused, and more in tune with your body, your husband, your friends and family, and life in general.

CHAPTER 8—HUMBLING YOURSELF UNTO THE LORD

Practical Advice for Couples Struggling with Infertility

Because couples face so many "unknowns" when they are trying to accept infertility issues, they need to remain a team. Marnie Deaton wrote the article, "Practical Advice for Infertile Couples" that I believe includes advice well worth heeding. She and her husband were childless for the first six years of their marriage. She says that besides experiencing unexpected, heart-wrenching spiritual battles, there were other situations that occurred for which they could have planned. Unfortunately their inexperience left them unprepared for much of what they faced.

Deaton says, *"the following advice may spare you some of the heartache we endured. As you realize that childbearing might not be as easy for you as it is for other couples, you would be wise to do some planning to protect yourselves:"*

1. Decide together who are the 'safe' people in your circle with whom you can share your struggle. I made the huge mistake of asking for prayer during a church service. We truly appreciated people's prayers, but some people in the congregation could not see us again without inquiring about our infertility. Each week they offered to pray for us, but in retrospect, it would have been better if we had selected a few people to ask for prayer.

2. Decide together how you will answer the question, *'So, why don't you have any children yet?'* Only God knows why people ask this, but they do and you have to be prepared for it. This question will hit you like a bus if you don't expect it and don't have a clear, well-thought-out answer in mind – an answer that, incidentally, is nearly impossible to find. I had the best results by simply saying, *'Unfortunately, we have not been blessed with children.'*

3. On that note, realize that you are going to have numerous chances to forgive people in the days ahead. People will tell you to 'just relax,' to gain or lose weight, to eat certain foods, and they may even joke that you and your husband must not 'know what you are doing.' They may pat your stomach and say they are praying for you. They may offer unsolicited advice. How should you deal with such people? I tried revenge, stewing, and bitterness, but the best response is forgiveness.

4. Consider not attending church on Mother's and Father's Days. One year, we accidentally attended church on Father's Day. To begin the service, our pastor invited all the fathers to stand. I will never forget my husband's expression as he looked at the floor while all the men around him stood up.

It was one of the worst moments of my life, and I cried buckets of tears for the rest of the service.

5. Find another infertile friend to confide in and support. No one can understand how painful infertility is unless they have been through it. If you are unaware of other infertile couples, you may consider finding a friend on the Internet. Trying to explain your situation to parents of growing families will only result in frustration.

6. Find other childless couples to have fun with. If you can't find other infertile couples, find some empty nesters or get involved in a youth group. In other words, find other people who are not parents to spend time with. If everyone in your church has children, find a new church. We should have done this. There were no young, childless couples in our church and Sundays were nearly unbearable. Looking back, I shouldn't have put myself through that. Sunday became an exercise in endurance rather than a time of worship.

7. Think of yourselves as a complete family unit. I learned toward the end of our infertility journey that God called creation 'good' after Adam and Eve met and before they had children. It helped me to remember that God thought of our marriage as good and complete, even without children. Realize that true legacy lies in passing on your values, love for God, and upright character, not your genes.

8. Remind yourself that, though infertility brings with it nearly unendurable pain, yours is not the worst situation in the world. As difficult as it is to face each day with empty arms, consider how painful it would be for a small child to go to bed alone each night without a parent to tuck him in, to watch over him, and to help him make it through the coming days. When I learned that thousands of children around the world were available for adoption, I began to count my blessings. I thank God each day for my parents.[11]

Another helpful hint comes from the August/September 2002 *Stepping Stones* newsletter, in which the unidentified author shares a way that couples can communicate without "beating a horse to death" so to speak.

"The 'Twenty Minute Rule' is a simple technique that allows a couple to talk about infertility or pregnancy loss, without allowing the subject to dominate and threaten the relationship. Here's how it works: Having discussed their infertility often and in depth in the past, the couple agrees that if one of them brings up an infertility-related subject, they will discuss it for 20 minutes but no longer. When this rule is skillfully applied, both spouses

benefit. She has his attention for a full 20 minutes instead of becoming frustrated because he is only listening with one ear. He benefits because he knows it is not going to be an all-night discussion. Best of all, they have the rest of the evening to talk about other topics and enjoy other activities."[12] Chapter 10 also includes practical marital advice.

Being Prepared for Insensitive Remarks and Suggestions

In the early stages of my encounter with infertility I was traveling for business a lot and normally the person seated next to me on the plane would try to make small talk. Inevitably their first questions would be:

"Are you married?"
"Yes," I replied.
"How long?" they queried.
"Six years," I responded.
"Do you have children?" they continued.

There I sat pondering my next answer. If I said *"no,"* I usually got the *Oh, she's too selfishly wrapped up in her career for a family* look, or the *Oh poor baby, she's probably sinned and this is her punishment* glare. Perhaps those people weren't judging me and I was blowing these scenarios out of proportion, nonetheless, I sat their feeling cold as ice, ashamed, and frustrated.

The problem is most people just assume that once you marry, you'll settle down and raise a family. This is true for some, but not for all of us. Some of us want to utilize our college educations for a while. Some women are very wise to spend time solidifying their marriages and the covenant they made with their husbands before talking about bringing children into the equation. And then there are those of us, who set out for pregnancy and our periods continue to devastate us month after month.

Truly, I know how you feel and I know the things you would like to say (and do), to people when they offer cruel remarks and insensitive suggestions. It is especially difficult when they are unsolicited! I mean how would they feel if I was sticking my nose into their personal life? Just who do they think they are? I'll tell you who they are: they are children of God just like you and me and we MUST treat them with the kindness and sensitivity that *they need to learn.*

By being prepared, there is less chance you'll be caught off guard and subsequently lash out at people. Marnie Deaton offered her pre-rehearsed response in the previous section. Here are a few ways that I personally found successful:

1. When making small talk with a stranger and the dreaded *Do you have children?* question came up, I had two *predetermined* answers to give. Either I said, "*I do not have children yet*" if it was a person who it seemed safe to have a further conversation with, or when it was a complete stranger, I said, "*No, how about you?*" That way the emphasis was back on them and we all know how people love to talk about themselves and their families.

2. Now and then when I ran into someone who knew of my situation and they seemed legitimately curious or interested, I tried to educate them on the *subject, not by personal story*. The reason I did that, is because in many cases, they were asking because their neighbor, or their friend, or their sister-in-law had the same problem and they didn't know how to talk to her. Ooccasionally the person I was talking with had been trying for several years and needed encouragement and guidance.

3. If you are a teacher, Sunday school leader, coach, piano instructor, tutor, or daycare facilitator, consider saying this when asked

"So, do you have any kids?"
"*Yes, I have 22!*"

That reply will easily seguay into your career or your interests instead of your personal life.

4. Christine said when the question came up her husband jokingly ended potentially on-going conversations quickly by saying they were still "practicing" or that they had been trying for several years. Irene got to the point that when people harrassed her about having children, she told them she didn't want kids (even though she did).

5. Ruth struggled with secondary infertility for 15 years. She says that questions such as "*Is he your only child?*" still sting, but she has chosen to answer this way: "*He is my only child, but not by choice. When God gave him to me, he gave me five in one! He is the most awesome kid!*" Another friend of mine answers this question by saying, "*Yes, we would really like to have* *another child, however our daughter's birth was a miracle and we're not sure if we will be able to have another child."* As you can see, when you memorize your predetermined answers, it's easier to be kind, forgiving and humble when you're put on the spot.

Part of being prepared involves taming that wicked "tongue" we talked about in Chapter 6. In the Book of James, Chapter 3, verses 1a through 10 (NLT) we are taught the following (notice this is directed to men too!): *"Dear brothers, don't be too eager to tell others their faults, for we all make many mistakes...*

If anyone can control his tongue, it proves that he has perfect control over himself in every other way. We can make a large horse turn around and go wherever we want by means of a small bit in his mouth. And a tiny rudder makes a huge ship turn wherever the pilot wants it to go, even though the winds are strong.

So also the tongue is a small thing, but what enormous damage it can do. A great forest can be set on fire by one tiny spark. And the tongue is a flame of fire. It is full of wickedness, and poisons every part of the body. And the tongue is set on fire by hell itself, and can turn our whole lives into a blazing flame of destruction and disaster.

Men have trained, or can train, every kind of animal or bird hat lives and every kind of reptile and fish, but no human being can tame the tongue. It is always ready to pour out its deadly poison. Sometimes it praises our Heavenly Father, and sometimes it breaks out into curses against men who are made like God. And so blessing and cursing come pouring out of the same mouth. Dear brothers, surely this is not right!"

By being prepared you won't have an issue to forgive. However, if an offence occurs, forgiving others does more good for you than it does for them. Try to be patient with your friends and relatives (*men [and women] who are made like God*).

Attending Child-Centered Occasions

Looking back, I did everything wrong when I was struggling with infertility. As you can see by the examples I have shared, if there was a right thing to do, I did the opposite. IF I did one thing right, I believe it was attending baby showers. Now, don't freak out; that was the right thing for ME to do. I had to surrender my personal fears, tears, aches, frustrations and disappointments for what? Three hours? I did that out of true happiness for my friends and family. Was it fun? No, it was long, drawn out and the games drove me crazy because I never knew the answers!

On the other hand, when I counsel women, I tell them that if they feel there's a chance they could end up making a scene, or saying something they'll regret, or ruining the party, then by all means DO NOT GO! Think of your wedding day. It was *your* day, you were the princess and if someone would have spoiled it, that's all you would remember about that special day.

I appreciate the honesty Allison shares about her feelings on this subject: *"Today was one of the most burdensome days of my three and a half years with infertility. I was to attend my cousin's baby shower, at a location approximately two and a half hours away. I left immediately after church in order to arrive on time for the shower. About fifteen minutes into the trip, I realized I was truly dreading this shower.*

What was I dreading? I was genuinely thrilled for my cousin. I honestly could not wait to meet the new baby and be a part of his life... so much potential in such a little boy. Yet, I still feared this shower.

When I gave it more thought, I realized why it was going to hurt. My entire family would be there oohing and aahing over cute baby items, joking about the burdens of pregnancy, and sharing their parental joy. This was my dream. It was this dream that I was looking forward to my entire life – sharing the pregnancy bond and parenting experiences with my family. But now, I was to witness this dream being lived by someone else. I was going to be a mere observer of my own dream.

My heart sank, I felt nauseated, and tears clouded my vision. I pulled off to the side of the road and I decided to turn back. Back to my husband's arms... back to where I knew I could show emotion without feeling weak or embarrassed. I realized that my pain was not simply going to occur at the shower—it was surrounding me. By attending the shower, I was actually trying to avoid the very thing I could not escape.

That decision to turn back was crucial. It was the moment when I first recognized that no matter how much you trust the Lord, the blows of life still hurt. Just because I am a Christian does not mean I am immune from feeling immense sorrow. Though our pain can be great, Christ has provided us with the grace to face our struggles. I have learned that grace can give us joy in the midst of our infertility. But grace, as spectacular as it is, does not stop life from hurting. Grace does, however, provide the hope needed to get through the pain.

My decision to turn the car around was not one of cowardice. It was the

CHAPTER 8—HUMBLING YOURSELF UNTO THE LORD

bravest decision I have ever made with respect to my infertility. The action of turning back meant I could no longer run away from the pain – I had to acknowledge its presence and face it. Today I turned back and found joy in Christ, as I faced the pain of life head on." [13]

I could brave my way through baby showers, however Mother's Day was the day of the year that caused me devastation. I absolutely hated that day. I loathed the insult I felt when at Sunday's service our pastor asked all the mothers to stand for acknowledgment. I despised the looks of pity I received from those who were aware of my situation. I abhorred going out to eat and seeing all of the mothers wearing corsages and toting their wee ones.

Looking back I realize that all those years of torment were unnecessary. I should have stayed home! You should consider avoiding anything that may make you sin on that day (or any day for that matter). If you attend church and sit there steaming or crying, and you can't listen to the sermon, or interpret the lyrics to the worship songs, realize that your eyes are off God and sin has prevailed.

Instead of feeling like the only one left out, put the focus on others. If you know someone who's lost their mother recently, ask if you can spend time with them that day. If you know of a couple that has undergone miscarriage or pregnancy loss, think about sending them a card or even flowers. Stop and think of the people in your world who have had an abortion or given their child up for adoption. Perhaps you could surprise them with an uplifting phone call. I try to call all of my infertile friends on Mother's Day because I want them to know I care about them and their feelings.

If you and your husband prefer to remain at home that day, plan ahead and rent some movies and prepare your favorite meal together. Be sensitive to the fact that your husband might not want to spend the day with you. Sometimes men have a hard time being around their wives when they are hurting because they want to "fix" their wife's pain and that is impossible for the most part.

One great regret I have from my 10-year struggle is that I focused on my dislike for Mother's Day and forgot all about my own mother. My mother is my best friend and I admire and love her dearly, yet I took her for granted. I dearly regret that mistake. I also have two mother-in-laws, two sister-in-laws who had children, as well as friends who were mothers and I focused on my pain and forgot to recognize their special day. Please avoid this mistake. If you have a good relationship with your mother, mother-in-law, grandmothers, aunts, etc., spend time focusing on them.

Handling Child-Centered Holidays

John and Sylvia Van Regenmorter have experienced infertility first hand. They offered suggestions for holiday "do's" and "don'ts" in the December 2000/January 2001 issue of *Stepping Stones* newsletter for which they are the editors: *"For those of us who are infertile, the holiday season, especially Thanksgiving, Christmas, and New Year's, can be a difficult time of the year.*

Each of these special days provides a wonderful opportunity for togetherness, thankfulness, and reflection. But for couples facing infertility issues, these holidays can also be painful reminders.

While many people around us give thanks for children, our homes remain childless. A Christmas celebration can be bittersweet when Grandma smiles at your sister's kids, and says, 'I love my grankids—I hope I have a lot more.' New Year's can be a solemn reminder of the passing of time and the failure to reach a cherished goal.

For those living with secondary infertility, the holidays become a pointed reminder that your one child has grown another year older without the companionship of a littler brother or sister. Couples who have faced pregnancy losses or an infant's death are reminded that there is no little one with whom to share the joy of Christmas morning.

There is no magic formula or wonder-working pill that can heal the hearts of couples who have no baby to hold during the holidays. But by proactively planning in advance for holiday hurdles, you can be better prepared for handling the hurts.

You may, in fact, discover some creative ways to have fun and celebrate the reason for the season." For the sake of space, I will shorten each suggestion significantly, therefore, to receive complete advice, go to step@bethany.org:

Do: Try to spend time with those who will leave you energized, not depleted.

Don't: Spend too much time with people who will add to your pain.

Do: Be selective about family gatherings if they have proven in the past to be too much to bear. If you must attend, consider arriving just in time for dinner and leaving early.

Don't: Feel that you have to 'tough it out' to the bitter end. Be selective about which family gatherings to attend.

Do: Start your own family traditions.

Don't: Assume that all of the old traditions will fulfill your new needs.

Do: Remember that it is okay to shed a tear and experience some sadness, but don't live there.

Do: Accept the reality that you cannot escape entirely. No matter how you play it, the holidays are going to bring some pain.

Don't: Deny the reality of these feelings or feel guilty about having them. Learn to recognize your feelings as legitimate emotions of loss and grief, [the grieving process is covered in the next chapter]. Don't try to argue yourself into believing that 'everything is fine,' and that you can carry on 'business as usual' during the holiday season.

Do: Follow the example of Jesus who said, 'For even the Son of Man did not come to be served, but to serve.' Reach out to others in need.

Don't: Close the door to positive feelings that come from helping others in need. Don't dwell on what you have not been given to the point that you lose sight of what you have received—namely, the privilege of knowing the 'good news of great joy that will be for all the people.'

On that note, if being around children is enjoyable to you, how about dressing up as the Easter bunny and surprising special children in your life at Easter? Perhaps your husband would entertain the thought of being Santa Claus at a family reunion. You two could even dress up as pilgrims and act out a short skit for neighborhood children. These ideas let the "kid" in you enjoy children during the holidays.

I would like to add that family and friends who have not experienced infertility, don't understand how you feel until you let them know. They should be made aware of your feelings in advance.

Dealing With Christmas

Christmas time is a wonderful season. I looked forward to spending time with my parents and immediate family to the point that I do not recall experiencing great sadness during my conflict with barrenness. Sure, I would have rather been baking cookies with my little girl, or decorating the tree with my sweet little boy. Somehow, I kept my focus on giving to others, enjoying family, and celebrating Christ's birth.

Some women feel just the opposite. We all know that Christmas is hectic and adding the stress of infertility can cause great anxiety. Family traditions and expectations can be overwhelming to some. I know of a woman who thoroughly enjoyed Christmas *before* her struggle with infertility, but afterward she found it depressing because the focus is mainly on children.

She tried to focus on the spiritual celebration but it was difficult for her because the focus is on pregnant Mary and Baby Jesus. She felt that because Christ came as a baby, she couldn't get past the baby focus in carols about "the newborn King," "Holy Infant so tender and mild," "this is the night of our dear Savior's birth," and "for unto us a Child is born."

If you are dealing with the same issues, consider the following advice so Christmas will be "merry" again:

1. When I stopped and thought about it, I spent every Christmas with my parents during the infertility journey. I couldn't bare the thought of waking up to an empty Christmas tree on Christmas morning; so being with family was comforting. Once my brothers had children, I enjoyed putting milk and cookies out for Santa with them. Seeing their smiling faces on Christmas morning was sheer pleasure.

2. When Christmas cards come brimming with family pictures and updates, do not allow your self to compare. Remind yourself that Jesus loves you as you are.

3. Furthermore, you don't have to have children to send out Christmas cards and updates; your friends and family love you and want to hear about your year. I advise you to keep depressing talk about your situation to a minimum. Yet subtly asking for prayer is a great idea.

4. Instead of focusing on Christ's life as a baby, study Christ's life as an adult.

5. Purposely focus on the real meaning of Christmas, not on how difficult this season may be for you.

6. If you don't plan to spend the holidays with relatives, do not allow yourselves to feel guilty about your decision. If you have had a recent loss, you may especially need that grieving period at home. However, if grieving will spiral the two of you into depression, carefully choose special loved ones to visit.

7. Consider making special plans with your immediate family. Take a trip, have a romantic dinner, watch old movies, get scrapbooks and home movies out to share with your children if you have them.

8. Consider "adopting" a needy family for Christmas. You can provide them with a Christmas meal or gifts. If you have a child, be sure to include them in the gift purchasing and delivering.

9. If you have a child, consider having a birthday party for Jesus. We put up

CHAPTER 8—HUMBLING YOURSELF UNTO THE LORD

balloons and banners, we decorate a cake and the children sing "Happy Birthday" and blow out candles, and we have a fun activity planned. Afterward, the children watch a kid's video depicting the story of Christ's birth. Sometimes we instruct party attendees to bring a gift and then we deliver those gifts to a single mother or needy family.

10. If you do attend family gatherings, consider arriving late and leaving early. Be sure to sit down and discuss as a couple what your feelings and plans for the holidays are in advance. Don't make your friends and family guess what you can handle—let them know in advance.

11. Make a point to reach out to others. You could serve food at a homeless shelter [I did this at Thanksgiving and it was very rewarding], visit shut-ins or nursing homes, or volunteer at your church or another facility.

12. If Christmas carols bother you, focus on these two: "Joy to the World" and "O Come, O Come Emmanuel."

13. Invite other infertile couples or those who have lost babies over for a meal. I advise you to discuss the rules of discussion beforehand. Plan to play cards or games, play music or watch a movie, and try to keep the evening light hearted and joyful.

14. It helped me to remain busy at Christmas time. Buying gifts kept me "other-oriented," baking for neighbors did too, and decorating the house with lights kept the Spirit of Christmas alive.

15. Attending church during the Advent season and especially the Christmas service truly helped me keep my mind on Christ's birthday.

In conclusion, Christmas isn't just about traditions, carols and turkey dinners; it's about a birthday that changed the fate of all mankind. When times are difficult at your house, force your mind to focus on that and show God your gratitude and adoration through your attitude and actions.

Childless at Christmas

"Christmas is the light that shines
In children's eyes," they say,
And often I feel such a void
In our home on Christmas day.

I'd love to take such loving care
To choose each special toy;
No sacrifice would be too great
To bring our dear child joy.

Then suddenly I see myself-
The child beneath the tree,
And after awesome sacrifice
My father watches me.

With great anticipation
Which gift will I like best?
But I'll accept just one thing
I kick away the rest.

Oh, Father God, forgive me
For my stubborn, selfish ways.
Teach me. Lord, to trust you ever
And to always offer praise.

By Lynn Campbell Behnke[14]

"Look after each other so that not one of you will fail to find God's best blessings. Watch out that no bitterness takes root among you, for as it springs up it causes deep trouble, hurting many in their spiritual lives." **Hebrews 12:15 (NLT)**

Chapter Nine–Opening Your Mind to Other Plans God Has for You

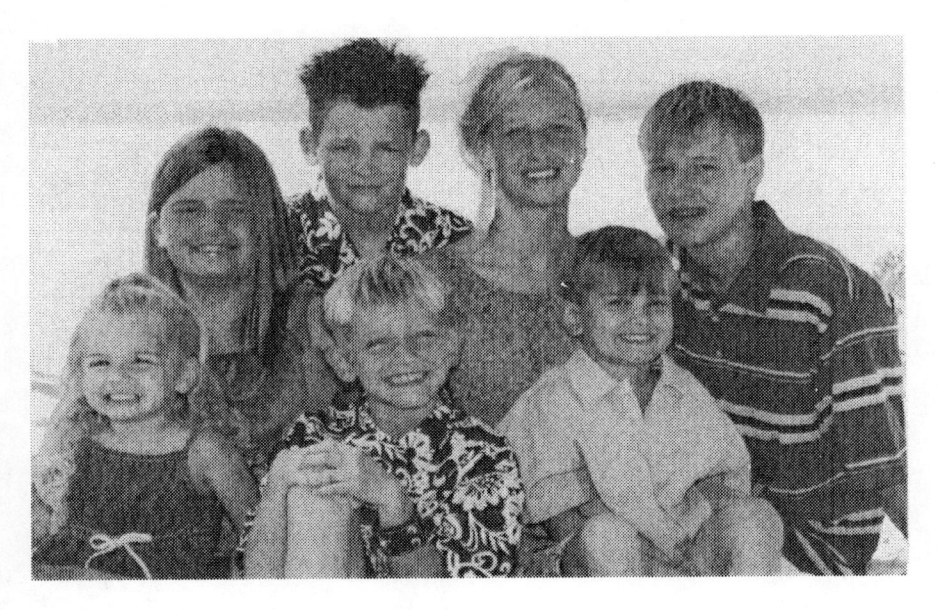

Shawn and Michelle's children: (Back row l to r) Alli, Brennan, Katia, John (Alosha), (front row) Abigail, Luke and Andrew

-Dealing with Pregnancy Loss
    Advice for Your Family and Friends
-Enlightening Family and Friends about Infertility
-Talking Before You Test
    What to Expect from Infertility Tests
    What to Expect from Advanced Procedures
-Considering Adoption
    What to Consider Before You Adopt
    Considering Foster Care

Chapter Nine–Opening Your Mind to Other Plans God Has for You

1. If you have experienced pregnancy loss, do you feel God understands the depth of your pain? Yes or No? (If you haven't gone through this pain, go on to question number 6.)

_____
_____
_____

2. Please describe the ways you cope with your loss:
_____
_____
_____

3. Please describe the ways your husband copes with his loss:
_____
_____
_____

4. Do you believe the child(ren) you have lost are in heaven with God right now? Yes or No?

5. List the people who have been supportive during your loss:

_____

_____

_____

Make sure to thank them.

6. If you have, or are considering infertility testing, have you sat down and talked with your husband about ramifications including cost, time, personal intrusion, ethical, and moral issues? Yes or No?

7. Have you and your husband determined how far you would go when it comes to testing? For instance, how do you both feel about In Vitro Fertilization? Do you have a "Plan B" if "Plan A" fails?

_____

_____

_____

8. When I say the words "foster care" and "adoption," what are the first thoughts that come into your mind?

_____

_____

_____

9. If I asked your husband this same question, what do you believe his responses would be?

_____

_____

_____

CHAPTER 9—OPENING YOUR MIND TO OTHER PLANS GOD HAS FOR YOU

10. Please describe your anxieties regarding testing, advanced procedures, adoption and foster care (if you have any):

_____

_____

_____

11. If the Lord leads you down the adoption path, would you consider this His wonderful plan for you or would this be an obligatory "second prize?" Please explain your feelings:

_____

_____

_____

Recommended Reading:

2 Chronicles 6:33, 39
Psalm 30:5, 34:18, 90:10, 138:7-8
Romans 8:17, 28
Galatians 6:2, 9

Job 11:16-20, 17:9
Proverbs 25:20
2 Corinthians 1:3-4
James 1:27, 5:16b

Look up these verses and fill in the blank:

Hebrews 10:36: *"You need to persevere so that when you have done the _____ of God, you will receive what he has promised."*

Galatians 6:2: *"Carry each other's _____, and in this way you will fulfill the law of Christ."*

"Why is Life so Unfair?"
Answer #8—A barren womb opens your mind to other plans God has for you... plans to prosper you in ways other than your own.

Chapter 9–Stacie's Story

I had to grow up quickly. I met my husband when I was 16-years-old and I knew the day I met him that I would marry him. Two years later I graduated from high school, turned 18, started planning our wedding, and found out I was pregnant. Brian's parents insisted we marry immediately. So, two weeks later I became a bride.

I had a very difficult pregnancy and was not sure of how to be a good wife. However, once the severe morning sickness passed our son was born. When Andrew was two months old I developed postpartum depression and had to be hospitalized. I could not take care of myself, much less my son.

When I was released, I learned my husband had moved in with his folks and they were taking care of Andrew. They had such a fear that I would hurt the baby, so they never left me alone with him. I remember one night I heard him cry, so I got up to give him a bottle and Brian's mother told me to go back to bed. She stated that she had everything under control and I was not needed. I was emotionally fragile and could not stand up for myself, or Andrew at the time. Walking back to my room with tears on my face, I felt that I had just lost him forever.

I had. We decided, with the agreement of my therapist, to look into putting Andrew up for adoption. When a friend of the family heard we were thinking of this option they spoke with a couple in our area. This couple had been trying for seven years to conceive and after a few conversations with them, Brian and I felt this was the right choice for Andrew. They picked him up on January 21, 1992—he was six months old.

Two years later we were given a second chance to have a child. In June of 1993, I discovered that once again I was pregnant. My mother was excited, but Brian's parents thought I was not mentally stable enough to have any more children. With the arrival of our daughter, Stephanie, it seemed all the past baggage seemed to slip away and my in-laws were happy for us. I suffered no effects of postpartum depression and I consider her my miracle baby to this day.

Almost a year and a half later, I gave birth to Matthew, a very large,

CHAPTER 9—OPENING YOUR MIND TO OTHER PLANS GOD HAS FOR YOU

strong baby boy. He was so amazing; at four-hours-old he lifted his head and looked at me for a few seconds. He loved to eat and he loved his sister. We felt that God had given us the perfect family. With the urging of Brian's parents we decided to get my tubes tied.

Wednesday, July 17, 1996, dawned like every other day. By 9:00 a.m. the kids were ready to be taken to their daycare. Brian and I dropped off Matthew and Stephanie, and set out to run our errands. Little did we know that would be the last time we would see our son alive. When we got home at 5:00 p.m. there was a message on the answering machine saying, 'Hi, it's Mom. There is something wrong with Matthew. You need to get to the daycare right away.' As we turned the corner it felt like we were moving in slow motion.

We immediately saw a fire truck, an ambulance and a police car. We ran into the daycare hoping that everything would be all right. The provider ran up to me saying, 'I am sorry, so sorry.' I pushed her aside and stepped into the living room. There were men in blue uniforms all over the room. As I was walking towards a group of them I heard, 'Here comes the mother.' Just as I reached the group a paramedic stepped aside to reach for something, and there was my baby.

It took a moment for the scene in front of me to register. He was lying on the coffee table with three paramedics working on him. Matthew was so blue and lifeless. There was a mask on his face as a paramedic forced air into his lungs, and his clothing was lying in tatters at his sides. A large paramedic was pumping his tiny chest. The paramedic's hands looked so big next to the small infant, yet they seemed to be ever so gentle. I watched another paramedic putting an IV into his head. I wanted to run to him pick him up and hold him, but something held me back.

Our son died of SIDS (Sudden Infant Death Syndrome), a silent killer for many babies. We chose to hold him and say our good byes. I remember praying that God would wake him and he would cry for me. It was then I realized he was gone forever. We would go home to an empty crib and broken hearts.

Since that day in 1996 when we buried Matthew, we have longed for more children. We've gone through great lengths including IVF, AI, a failed adoption, reconstructive surgery (to restore my fallopian tubes), more tests, more fertility drugs, gastric bypass surgery, taking a break, and through it all I've experienced four miscarriages.

I am 30 years old and I have been through so much. I could have never gone through this without God. Of course it's been rough and I don't understand His will for me, but I think I'm finally at a point of surrender. Brian and I are looking into foster care and adoption and we are just letting Him steer the course. We've still got our precious Stephanie and our home is open to more children—if it is His will.

> **"Trust in the Lord with all your heart and lean not on your own understanding…"** **Proverbs 3:5**

Dealing with Pregnancy Loss

Although I still feel the "sting" of never being pregnant, never experiencing life within me, never giving birth or breast feeding, never seeing a baby with *my* eyes and *my* fingers, I have thanked God repeatedly that I did not become pregnant and then experience miscarriage or loss. I can't even think about it without tears welling up in my eyes. To Stacie, and to you my dear friends who have gone through that kind of devastation and grief, I extend my most sincere apologies.

As you can see from Stacie's story, it's so hard to understand God's reasons for removing a child from this world. I guess it is part of the trial – the part that teaches faith and perseverance.

Nancy S. Kingma, BSN, RN, is a Bereavement Coordinator at Spectrum Health in Grand Rapids, MI. In an article she wrote titled "The Death of a Baby: How Couples Cope," she says with the death of a baby, a couple shares the loss of their dreams and a precious part of themselves and their future.

Kingma said that although the couple may feel very connected to each other in the first days and weeks after their baby's death, it is important for them to realize that grief is very personal and individual. Even when a couple has been together for many years, they most likely will not grieve in the same way. Both partners are hurting, but because of different influences and expectations in their lives, they may be experiencing and showing grief in different ways.

"The woman," she says, *"may desire to sit, cry, and talk continually about her baby."* She explains further: *"Sadness overwhelms her. She may experience insomnia, nightmares, and either loss of appetite or overeating. Disruptions in life may bring tears, rage, or tension. She may feel abandoned and have the need to be held and comforted rather than have sexual intimacy.*

CHAPTER 9—OPENING YOUR MIND TO OTHER PLANS
GOD HAS FOR YOU

The man *may bury himself in his work, which brings comfort and stability to his life. It is not uncommon for the man to involve himself in strenuous physical activity such as playing racquetball or chopping wood. He may not want to talk about the baby because he is afraid of 'breaking down.' He might worry about the intensity of his partner's grief and may attempt to help her 'cheer up' or 'move on' with life."*

Kingma says it is not uncommon for a man to delay his grieving until he knows his partner is "handling things" better. While the man may feel uncomfortable hugging and holding his partner, sexual intimacy may bring emotional closeness for him.

Because each spouse grieves differently, it is hard for him or her to understand each other. She notes a woman may believe her partner did not love the baby as much as she did because he does not talk about the baby or cry with her. The man may believe he is a failure because he is not able to protect his partner and make her life happy again.

At a time when it would be beneficial for the couple to be communicating about their loss and its effect on their lives, they may feel estranged and isolated. This lack of communication may add further stress to the relationship, she adds.

According to Kingma, *"There is no simple way for a couple to deal with grief and loss. To recognize some of the different ways each grieves can help the couple understand each other and help each other grieve. Perhaps the best course of action is patience and openness."*

Kingma offers the following advice to couples experiencing pregnancy loss:

1. Attempt to accept each other's differences and limitations.
2. Give your spouse the time he or she needs to grieve.
3. Avoid blaming each other.
4. Focus on the love you have for one another. Go on a date at least once a week and concentrate on your relationship.
5. Plan a special time of holding, caring, and recognizing that your love continues, even in your grief.
6. Spend time talking about your baby and the loss you have experienced.
7. Slow your life down as much as possible. Attempt to put off any major decisions in your life. (Change may make the grief more intense.)
8. If you feel you need help, get it. Seeking assistance is not a sign of weakness. It is an act of love toward yourself and your partner.

9. Above all, pray for each other and with each other as you bring your pain to the Lord. Don't be afraid to share your emotions, questions, and anger with Him. He can handle it. In time, through quiet and simple ways, He will begin the healing process in your hearts and lives.[1]

Read how Marilyn describes her loss: *"I always wanted three children. I come from a family of five and so does my husband, so I just had it in my head that, that's how it was going to be —three children. When we started out, I had a miscarriage. I started spotting the day I was going to announce my pregnancy at work. The drive to the doctor was the worst. What got me through that loss was the knowledge that I **did** get pregnant.*

Later, we had a daughter and then when I was pregnant with my son, I started spotting again, this time at three months. I was terrified. That was harder to take than the miscarriage, but thankfully, Matthew was fine. If I could offer any advice, I would remind women that if they have a pregnancy loss, try to see the positive side that you did get pregnant. Not everyone gets that far. Be aware that it's not as easy to get pregnant as it seemed when we were young girls." I find it interesting that God answered Marilyn's prayers for three children. She has two of them in her household and He has the other one in His.

When Marilyn started bleeding, she was instructed to go to the hospital so her doctor could ascertain if she was losing the baby. Janet describes this process and what happens when you arrive at the hospital: *"Although I had two miscarriages, I only had a **D & C (Dilatation & Curettage)** with one of them. I was 10 weeks along and woke up to bloody sheets. Once it got heavier, I decided to call the doctor and was told to go to the emergency room where he would meet me. After registering, I was taken to a treatment room where they began a series of tests.*

They took my blood to determine the HCG (Human Chorionic Gonadotropin) level and see if the level was falling – this would determine whether the pregnancy was failing or not. They also did an internal exam to determine the amount of blood loss, the position of the uterus, and if the cervix was open. Next, they performed an ultrasound to see if a heartbeat could be detected. If no heartbeat is detected, the level of HCG is dropping, and the cervix is open, this is usually a clear indication of miscarriage.

If you have this procedure, they will then determine the amount of blood you are losing. At this point they will determine whether to send you home or if a D & C is needed to help assist with the removal of the pregnancy lining to stop excessive bleeding. If surgery is required, it is considered an outpatient procedure. You will be wheeled into the surgery room with an IV and then put

CHAPTER 9—OPENING YOUR MIND TO OTHER PLANS GOD HAS FOR YOU

under general anesthesia. The surgery will last about an hour and the recovery takes about two hours. Although your heart will be heavy, your physical recovery will be very quick with minimal pain.

Generally, you will be sent home with a prescription for antibiotics and instructions to rest for a day or two. You will then have a follow-up examination in your OB office. He or she will examine you internally to make sure everything is healing correctly; they will check for infection and determine how you are doing emotionally. If all checks out, you will usually want to wait three months before trying to have a baby again."

If you have undergone the heartbreak of pregnancy loss, you may be feeling the way this honest, young lady felt: *"I'm kind of angry with God right now. I know I shouldn't be, but I am. Why would He do this to me? Why did I get pregnant after all this time just to miscarry? I am trying to figure it out, but the answers don't come. I suppose I will have to wait until I get to heaven to know for sure."*

Ruth shares an optimistic way that she views her losses: *"Not long after our fist miscarriage, two ladies from our church came to visit me, bringing with them a gift from the Ladies Sunday School class: a rosebush. I remember thanking them, and exclaiming how beautiful it was.*

After they left, I laughed at myself – it was February and the rosebush was certainly not beautiful at that season; it looked like a lifeless twig planted in a box! Yet I could see the picture of pink roses on the box, and I knew that someday, perhaps not this summer but next, it would bloom.

And then I realized... I was like that rosebush. Right then I felt like an old dead twig – my hopes, my dreams, had been snatched from me, leaving me feeling withered and barren and lifeless. In my journal I wrote: 'The Lord sees my life, and in His eyes it is becoming beautiful. Someday I will leaf out and bloom. Only God knows what sort of bloom that will be; perhaps I will give birth to a baby, perhaps a child will join our family through adoption, or perhaps the Lord wants me to give up my wishes for children and surrender to His alternate plan. I can't see 'the picture on the box' of my life, but God can. And I can rest in His loving care."[2]

I once read how another woman leaned on Proverbs 3:5 after her miscarriage. She said, *"I came to realize that God wasn't asking me if I understood what was happening in my life, but he was asking me if I trusted Him. God was saying to me 'You don't need to understand, you just need to trust me.'"*

I'm not sure I will ever fully understand God's reasoning for pregnancy loss. I believe it was meant to remain a mystery. However, I like to think that God was so in love with your children that He couldn't wait to have them in heaven with Him. He made sure they would never, ever experience pain, sorrow, sin or fear. In His fatherly fashion, He is holding and hugging them, He is playing ball and baking cupcakes with them, *until you arrive to join them.*

To The Child We Briefly Knew

As our child leaves this world,
There's so much that we don't know –
What she could have been, what she could have done,
If given a chance to grow.
We never knew her smile,
Or brushed her soft, dark hair,
We never kissed her wounded knee
Or chose what she would wear.
Our empty arms remind us
Of the place that she should be;
But somehow, though we don't know why,
You've taken her with Thee.

By Stephanie Garcia[3]

Advice for Your Family and Friends

When your loved one or friend goes through pregnancy loss, how do you handle it? I am the kind of person who avoids confrontation at all costs. It's difficult for me to pick up the phone and acknowledge people's losses, hurts and disappointments. I realize this might not seem like confrontation, but to me it's the unknown.

I find myself wondering, *how will they react when I call? Are they going to break down and cry? I can't handle tears! What if they are so upset that they take it out on me?* I tend to "what if" myself to the point that I put off the telephone calls indefinitely. I fear, that in reality, my silence says, *I don't care* to them.

CHAPTER 9—OPENING YOUR MIND TO OTHER PLANS GOD HAS FOR YOU

Sadly, this is how my family and I handled my brother and sister-in-law's miscarriage several years ago. I truly regret the fact that to avoid personal sadness and discomfort, we basically "swept the miscarriage" under the rug. Tears and sadness were avoided because they were considered signs of weakness. Looking back, if I had been in Justin and Marilyn's shoes, I would have been so hurt that my baby was not acknowledged as a once living soul. I feel that I owe all three of them an apology.

Perhaps in our silence we were trying to avoid "careless words," or maybe we were trying to save our own skins. Kathleen A. Massey wrote an article on this subject. She advises: *"Anyone dealing with infertility and miscarriage knows how often we're faced with an inappropriate question or comment from others. Most of us learn to live with it and try to answer with some sensitivity. Others get angry and respond cuttingly. Some will try to lighten the subject with humor. I usually try to answer the questions and correct the frequent misinformation in the hopes of saving another from a similar confrontation.*

On one occasion, when a woman said something I knew I'd have to forgive her for, the Lord whispered, 'careless words.' Suddenly I realized what He meant – at least as far as infertility and miscarriage are concerned: Careless words spoken to one who is hurting is an attempt to relieve the discomfort of the one speaking."

Massey explains that empathy and compassion for the hurting makes us want to say something. However, we often speak to relieve our own discomfort. We've all been in those awkward situations where we didn't know what to say and felt uncomfortable. In such cases, we usually avoid the situation or mumble some general response.

*"Please remember that **sometimes** the best response to a hurting person is silence."* She adds, *"When the Holy Spirit urges us to be silent, it means, 'be a good listener.' Most people needing the ministry of comfort require someone who will listen and acknowledge their pain. Most people in pain know that you don't have the answer. They just want to tell you about the situation with which they are dealing.*

The physical and emotional pain of three miscarriages was hard on me, and on all those who loved me. Most felt obligated to respond in some way. Though their responses were all motivated by love, some came across as careless words. Instead of listening to the Spirit, some people around me yielded to their need to respond. Those words hurt me and only added to my burden."

Massey shares these examples of **what not to say** to your hurting friend or loved ones:

- **You're still young; you'll have other chances.** Even if other children come along, it doesn't diminish the pain of losing this child. Besides, I have as much trouble getting pregnant as I do maintaining a pregnancy, so how do you know there will be another chance.
- **Don't give up. My aunt had four losses before finally carrying a child to term.** This means: be glad, it could be worse. Hurt isn't minimized by comparison. It's hard enough to work out my own grief without adding others' to it.
- **It's probably for the best.** Nature has a way of rejecting problem pregnancies. God has a way too! It's called healing. My God could have healed anything wrong with my child or me. He could also have not allowed me to get pregnant again, only to lose it. But He had something else in mind.
- **At least you have one!** My son is not a consolation prize. It is my joy and love for Justin that makes my longing for another child so strong. It will never lessen the pain of loss.

So, what should you do? *"Learn to listen to the Holy Spirit and follow His lead. If you don't hear anything, don't make something up. Just listen to the person and acknowledge the pain,"* Massey said. She also says it is very helpful for the hurting person if you are able to respond in these tangible ways:

1. Take them dinner.
2. Clean their house.
3. Hug or hold hands.
4. Let them cry; cry with them.
5. Care for their children to give them a day alone.
6. Take care of errands or grocery shopping.
7. Send flowers.
8. Remember the anniversary of a death with a card or phone call.
9. Pray for them.
10. Tell them you are praying for them.
11. Notify their church.

She concludes, *"In all ways, treat the loss of a pre-born child or a newly born child the same as if it were an older child."*[4]

CHAPTER 9—OPENING YOUR MIND TO OTHER PLANS
GOD HAS FOR YOU

Lorena expands on this advice by adding the following list of "do's" and "don'ts" specifically for friends and family of those who have undergone pregnancy loss:

Don't tell me, 'You can have another baby.' How do you know? Beside, I want this baby.

Don't tell me, 'At least it happened before it was born. It's not like you knew the baby.' I did know my baby. For the short time s/he was with me, I loved my baby with all my heart. I had hopes and dreams for this baby. I had names picked out and a theme for the nursery. I knew my baby was going to be a very special person.

Don't tell me, 'It's just one of those things.' It was not just 'one of those things' from my viewpoint. Miscarriage has had a devastating effect on my life, and making it sound as though it was an unimportant event does not lessen the impact.

Don't tell me 'it's common,' or 'it happens to a lot of women.' This happened to me, and all I want is to have my baby back.

Don't tell me, 'It was just a blob of tissue.' In my heart and in God's eyes, I know I was carrying a living being inside me from the moment s/he was conceived. Please don't trivialize my beliefs or that precious life.

Don't tell me, 'You should be over it by now.' Even though the physical effects may have subsided, I am still hurting emotionally. My child has died, and it takes much longer than a week or two to recover from that pain.

Don't tell me, 'You'll get over it.' The miscarriage was the death of my child. I will never 'get over it.' The pain and grief will eventually lessen, but I will always wonder what my child would have been like. Every should-have-been birthday, and every anniversary of the miscarriage will be a reminder.

Don't tell me, 'You should get pregnant again as soon as possible. That'll help.' Help what? I need time to grieve the baby I have lost. I can't even begin to think about getting pregnant again at this time.

Don't tell me, 'It won't happen again. The next time will be fine.' Again, how do you know? My second pregnancy ended in miscarriage also, even after doctors said there was no reason it wouldn't be successful the second time around.

Do listen to me when I want, or need, to talk about what I am going through.

Do be sensitive to the fact that I probably won't want to hear about your pregnant friend/neighbor/cousin/daughter, or about your new grandchildren or nieces or nephews for a while.

Do give me time to grieve. Some days I may need your shoulder to cry on after everyone else thinks I should be 'okay' by now.

Do understand that there are 'milestone days,' such as the expected due date of the time I should have felt the first kick, when I will be feeling the loss as deeply as when the miscarriage occurred. I will need your support then.

Do know that I am like any other person who has experienced the death of a loved one. I may not feel like talking when you come for a visit, or I may do things you may think inappropriate – such as clean the house– just to have something to do so I don't have to think. Be patient with me.

Do show caring to others who have experienced miscarriage. Treat their loss with the same respect and love you would give if they were suffering the death of any other loved one.

Do let those of us who are going through – or have gone through – miscarriage know that we are not alone. Send a note or make a phone call or let us know you're thinking of us, especially on those difficult 'milestone days.' Sometimes we feel that we're the only ones who remember, and it's nice to know that our baby was important to you too."[5]

Janet's husband, Edward, helped make the pain of her two miscarriages a little easier to bear by doing the following: *"My husband bought me a beautiful black hills gold cross pendant and had the dates of my miscarriages imprinted on the back. It helped that he acknowledged the importance of those dates."*

Janet recalls, *"He also sent me flowers on the first anniversary of my first miscarriage and wrote a note stating that this was from my little angel up above, and that my angel was doing just fine up in heaven. Talk about an emotional outburst in front of the deliveryman!! My charm bracelet sports two tiny crosses representing each of the angels I lost. And, our Christmas tree also has two beautiful cross ornaments that have dates engraved on the backs. It is a special time for me each Christmas as I hang them on the tree."*

As Lorena said, try not to place grieving deadlines on people. Connie said that many people expect you to get over a miscarriage or loss quickly. She says that many people don't seem to consider unborn children as "real," so they have less sympathy to offer. They seem to think that since you didn't have the baby and get attached to it that you'll get over the loss quickly. She adds, *"Nobody ever forgets their loss, but others seem to think the hurt just goes away after awhile. In reality, it is a lifetime of knowing you will never hold, get to know, or see what the future held for your child."*

Valerie told me that when she was at Bible study one day, all her friends crowded around one of the ladies whose child had recently died. They grieved with her and offered her encouragement and support. Not one person acknowledged the miscarriage that had just devastated Valerie's dreams. She and I agree that it seems that women who have miscarriages are taboo – nobody wants to be around them, so they just pretend like nothing happened. Please make a point to acknowledge miscarriage and pregnancy loss. If it is difficult to call or visit, consider sending a note or even flowers.

Last, if you have a baby and you're going to be around a woman who just lost a child or who has recently had a miscarriage, be considerate and have someone else hold your infant when she enters the room. Embrace her and comfort her *without* your newborn in your arms. She will let you know if she desires to hold your child or not.

Enlightening Family and Friends About Infertility

In the introduction I promised family and friends of infertile couples suggestions and advice. The previous section should help you when your loved ones experience pregnancy loss and this section is targeted to infertility in general.

Terry Willits, author of "How to Encourage an Infertile Friend," says that being infertile is very difficult and being the friend or family member of those who are infertile is also very difficult. She offers the following advice and steps you can take to be encouraging rather than unknowingly hurtful:

"You hurt for [your infertile friends or family members] and probably feel helpless, not knowing what to say or do to express your love and encourage them during this painful time in their lives. After personally experiencing five years of infertility, I can say with some authority, that many friends have done 'the right things' to encourage me, and many friends have (unknowingly) acted inappropriately," said Willits.

The following suggestions are intended to help you minister effectively – not offensively – to the one(s) you love. Willits says please keep in mind that these are general suggestions. Infertile couples experience various amounts of stress and pain in their lives. But one thing is certain – they are hurting. Extra sensitivity on your part can prevent you from causing your friends or family members additional pain, regardless of their stage of infertility.

She offers this warning before you continue: If you do have a friend or family member who is undergoing infertility, and you truly want to minister to them, you are about to embark on a very selfless adventure. It is one that God will honor and your friend will never forget. If you are willing to accept this mission, read on!

Steps You Can Take:

1. Pray diligently for your loved ones. Place a reminder (a photo or a note) where you will see it often. Pray that God will give you the wisdom to offer encouragement to your friend. James 5:16b says, 'The prayer of a righteous man is powerful and effective.' There truly is power in prayer, and your friend needs your prayers more than anything.

2. Drop your friend a note when the Lord places that person on your heart. Tell your friend that you love him/her, hurt for him/her, and are praying for him/her. Putting your feelings into written words can often be easier than expressing them orally. Notes from friends can be very effective – for they can be personal and express loving support without putting the recipient on the spot to respond. Trust God to inspire the timing of your notes.

3. Let your actions show your love. Give your friend a warm hug from time to time. Buy your friend something to make him/her feel special. Actions always speak louder than words.

4. Make time for your friend. Meet him/her for lunch. Get a sitter or neighbor to watch your children. The visit without children might benefit both of you. Your friend needs your undivided attention and encouragement.

5. Be understanding if your friend seems distant at times. If you have children or are expecting, it may be painful for your friend to be in contact with you. Remember, this is a season in your friend's life. If you have a strong relationship, your friendship will survive this time of testing and trial.

In Conversation…

If you are just getting to know someone, **do not ask if they have children**. If they do, more than likely, they will let you know, and if they don't, it's not your place to ask why not. At a rehearsal dinner recently, I was asked four times within five minutes if I had children. I wanted to crawl under the table and cry. A good alternative to asking about children is *'Tell me about yourself.'*

1. Think before you bring up the subject of infertility. Asking about someone's infertility depends a great deal on the depth of your friendship. If you are close friends, certainly ask from time to time how things are going.

CHAPTER 9—OPENING YOUR MIND TO OTHER PLANS
GOD HAS FOR YOU

Your friend will appreciate your concern. If it's not a good time to talk, he or she will let you know. Let your friend guide the conversation. Don't push. Likewise, if your friend is a casual acquaintance, he/she may prefer not to discus infertility. Take your clues from your friend.

2. Broaden the topics you discuss. It is inconsiderate to talk only about parenthood. Take your signals from your friend. If your friend is doing well and feeling strong, he/she will probably ask about your children. If your friend's period just started, or if she just heard about someone else's pregnancy, your words may trigger great discouragement.

3. Realize that jokes can be counter-productive. Comments like, *'Why don't you drink our water?'* or *'Do you want to borrow our kids?'* are simply unkind. If you feel awkward with the situation, it is better to say nothing. If you have never experienced infertility, do not say that you understand. Even if you have been through infertility, no two situations are identical. More than likely, all your friend wants is a listening ear. You can still be compassionate and minister without having to relate your life experiences to your friend.

About Giving Advice:

1. Do not offer advice unless your friend asks for it. Don't tell your friend that you stood on your head, went on vacation to the Bahamas, or bought your husband boxer shorts in order to get pregnant. She has probably tried it all and your advice is not helpful; it is hurtful. Such advice also suggests that achieving pregnancy is within one's control.

2. Avoid telling your friends to 'RELAX'. The 'R' word sends shivers up any infertile person's spine. This cliché' is offered as advice by many well-meaning friends. Studies show that 90 percent of infertility is due to medical problems in one or both mates (10 percent to unknown causes). Relaxing will not change one's medical condition. Telling a person to relax makes light of that person's situation. Once again, such advice implies that the person has control over his or her fertility. The last thing your friend needs is another reason to feel that he/she is a failure.

3. Do not suggest adoption as a means to a natural birth. Avoid comments like, 'Just adopt, then you will get pregnant.' Although adoption can be a wonderful option, it is no guarantee that one will someday conceive a biological child. Choosing to adopt is a very personal and private decision. Some couples are more sensitive than others regarding adoption. If your friend is considering adoption, he/she will bring it up.

Avoid Making Judgments:

1. Do not 'over spiritualize' infertility. Many infertile couples struggle with the false belief that they have done something wrong to deserve their fate, and they are unworthy of the 'reward from God' called children. Be careful not to reinforce this perception with comments like, 'Well, God must be trying to do this or that in your life' or 'you must not be ready for children or God would have given them to you.' As Christians, we need to avoid making such assumptions. No one truly knows the mind of God.

2. Do not stand in judgment of your friend's attempts to achieve fertility. Each couple has their own personal convictions regarding medical treatment. What is acceptable and appropriate for one couple may not be appropriate for another. Be careful not to criticize treatments.

Encourage Healing:

1. Put away your toolbox. Don't try to fix things. Just love your friend and listen. Allow your friend the freedom to express anger. As with all types of grief, there are stages, and anger is an important stage. Your friend's anger may be directed toward him/herself, others, and even God. The only path to healing is to recognize and express this anger without being condemned for such feelings.

Job was a man of faith, patience, and endurance, yet he complained freely and bitterly to God and his close friends in the midst of his incredible sorrows. Expressing anger was necessary to complete his emotional healing and to restore his relationship with God. Nothing heals anger faster than a response of unconditional love and acceptance.

2. Be patient with the 'pity party'. As with any trial in life, your friend may fall into the trap of ungratefulness and self-pity. Be patient. However, if this self-pity persists and you are very close to your friend, a gentle confrontation may be necessary. Seek God before you speak up. It is absolutely essential that your motivation be purely to minister and encourage your friend. (Consult Galatians 6:1 to check your motivation and your own spiritual condition before you confront your friend.)

CHAPTER 9—OPENING YOUR MIND TO OTHER PLANS GOD HAS FOR YOU

Pregnancy/Baby Showers/Childbirth:

1. Use tact when announcing your pregnancy. If your friend lives locally, either share your news alone, in person (not in public) or drop her a note. Tell your friend that you realize the news may be painful for her to hear. Reassure your friend of your love and continuing prayers. If your friend lives out of town, write her a letter. This will give her time and space to accept it and not be put on the spot for an immediate response.

2. If you're expecting a baby, use common sense. For example, it would be inappropriate to ask your friend about suggestions for baby names or nursery decor; to show your friend a sonogram photo; or to ask her to feel the baby kick. If your friend is interested, she will inquire.

3. If your friendship is very close and your friend has been going through infertility for a while, do not place her on an invitation list for your baby shower. Being in a room full of people who talk about babies for hours can be too overwhelming. Instead, call her and explain that you'd like to include her, but you do not want to cause her the least pain. A woman struggling with infertility often experiences false guilt if she is emotionally unable to attend her closest friend's baby shower. If she really wants to go, she'll let you know. Instead of attending the shower, suggest that you get together for lunch.

4. Ask your friend ahead of time how she wants to be told when the baby comes. Plan on someone other than you (the elated parent) announcing the birth of your child. It will be easier to hear the news from another family member or friend. The ball is now in your friend's court to respond.

Remember who is in control.

"Recognize that no matter how hard you try to encourage your infertile friend, our Heavenly Father is the only One who can truly give comfort, strength, hope, and peace," concludes Willits.[6]

Most people don't realize that certain occasions and holidays are very difficult for infertile couples. Family reunions, as well as gatherings at Thanksgiving and Christmas are difficult, children's birthday parties are especially hard to handle, and one of the most difficult occasions is Mother's Day.

Angie shares ways people have been sensitive to her regarding this occasion: *"On Mother's Day last year, I was very blessed to have two friends show me how much they cared about me. Both friends knew I get depressed during the week of Mother's Day. One friend sent me flowers and then stopped by later with a cookbook she knew I wanted. The other friend came to my door one afternoon sobbing. She had had a miscarriage several years earlier and she wanted me to have her baby when I got to heaven. I was speechless. This was a person who understood my pain and emptiness. She knew my arms would never be full on earth, so she wanted to fill them in heaven. She is a friend like no other.*

My two sisters have been constantly sensitive for as long as I can remember. One sister sent me flowers this past Mother's Day and the other called on Sunday to see how I was doing. They both are loving and supportive. When one of my sisters was pregnant with my niece, she never talked about her pregnancy unless I asked her. Even today, she doesn't talk about her daughter unless I ask questions. God has blessed me with two very sensitive sisters.

I am thankful for those times when I have been able to lean on the Lord because someone hurt me. I am also thankful for the times when others have been sensitive to my need for understanding or my feeling of emptiness. Their kindness brings me closer to the Lord.

There is no trick to being sensitive. It takes time and empathy. The world would be a better place if people would stop and think before they speak."[7]

When you know of a family with an only child, don't be too quick to judge them. There's a chance they are devastated that a second, full-term pregnancy eludes them. For instance, while teaching women with secondary infertility, Eileen has witnessed how secretive they tend to be for fear of seeming ungrateful for the child or children they've been blessed with. She says if they speak up about their disappointment, they seem complaining and never satisfied. Eileen adds, "*You have the group with no children who think, 'Shut up and get over it and count the blessing you already have.'*

Another group typically has two or more children and constantly reminds the woman with one how easy it was for them. Then there is the group that is completely clueless and say rude things to her about having only one child and they continually ask why she doesn't want more."

The woman (or couple) struggling with secondary infertility is stuck in the middle. They hear it from both sides. They are suffering and need to confide in people who won't judge them. You can be there to listen. You can use this information to help instead of hurt others.

Finally, please don't make a barren woman feel obligated to hold your

CHAPTER 9—OPENING YOUR MIND TO OTHER PLANS GOD HAS FOR YOU

baby or play with your children. You're not always doing her a favor. Let her ask you. Most of us experiencing the confusion and loneliness of infertility, feel like we are living a dirty secret. We often want to hide away and pretend like nothing bad is happening to us. Give us time and space. Be supportive and don't criticize our decisions. Celebrate our successes and be patient with us. The more you are aware of the intensity of our struggle, and the more you understand that we need your tolerance and support, the better friends we all will be.

> *"Carry each other's burdens, and in this way you will fulfill the law of Christ,"* **Galatians 6:2.**

Talking Before You Test

Whether or not you experience miscarriage or pregnancy loss, every couple who encounters infertility will get to a point when they need to consider seeking medical help. Chapter 2 contained a list of conditions to consider regarding when it's time to pursue infertility testing.

Again, I admit this is a big decision. Not only are you admitting a problem, you are opening yourselves up to embarrassing questions, humiliating procedures, some pain and discomfort, expense, and time. I really had no options left, so booking that first appointment with my gynecologist was my way of taking action.

Many couples have asked my opinion about the moral and ethical issues involved. I believe God gave us medical advances for a reason. For example, when our eyesight is blurred, we go to an optometrist for glasses. Seeking medical aid for infertility seems just as natural to me.

When you and your bridegroom are in the midst of making the decision whether or not to consider a professional opinion, here are some suggestions I would like you to keep in mind and to discuss amongst yourselves:

1. You would be wise to sit down with your husband and determine a list of "do's" and "don'ts" before you are up to your eyeballs in doctor's appointments, medical bills and big decisions. For example, this may sound cold, but you and your husband need to assess together how much money you can afford before testing.

2. You would be wise to check with your insurance company about their ability to cover procedures before you start. Our checkbook dictated when and what procedures were done and that's why the process took so long. This intensified my frustration because endometriosis (tissue that grows in places other than the uterus such as on the fallopian tubes or ovaries) was growing rapidly on a daily basis. Also, keep in mind, that if you want to consider adoption as an alternative, you must factor in those costs.

3. If there are procedures that make one or both of you uncomfortable, or that you disagree with morally, discuss this beforehand. Discuss your feelings about masturbation, pornography, pregnancy reduction and embryo reduction *before* they become an issue. These matters will very likely come up and it will help if you do your research beforehand (that includes Biblical research!).

4. Don't force your spouse to start or stop testing. I basically went through testing without my husband's emotional support and it ended up adding to my already mounting anxiety and resentment. I also made the decision to stop testing without consulting him and several years *later* my husband confessed to me that he wished I had at least tried Artificial Insemination or In Vitro Fertilization. This was news to me, because I never asked him.

5. Sit down with your doctor (I highly recommend that you see a fertility specialist and that you take the time to investigate his or her merits beforehand), and ask him or her to give you an honest evaluation of your likelihood of pregnancy. I hate to be the bearer of bad news, but they are more than happy to take your money as long as you are willing to give it. They basically do what you authorize, so have them give you a definite opinion of what tests should or should not be done in advance and when testing should be terminated.

6. Before seeing a specialist, my gynecologist suggested that I do preliminary testing on my own that would be useful to him. These tests included temperature charting, mucus testing and use of an ovulation predictor test kit. My gynecologist also had my husband's sperm tested for count, morphology and motility. So, when I approached the specialist, my charts, reports and results were helpful in establishing a plan of action.

7. Many of the couples I have spoken with made the decision to stop testing and then started again at a later date. Realize that this is okay. Typically, they become more educated on the services available and decide to take a chance while they are still young. Others have changed insurance carriers and are better prepared financially to exhaust all avenues of testing. Sometimes people just need a break. Testing can be discouraging, painful, humiliating and intrusive to one's marriage and personal life.

CHAPTER 9—OPENING YOUR MIND TO OTHER PLANS
GOD HAS FOR YOU

8. If you decide together that it's time to stop testing, don't let yourselves feel guilty that your desire to be parents wasn't great enough to be more aggressive in testing further. Guilt is a trap from the evil one. If he puts condemning or guilt-driven thoughts into your head, capture them, dispel them, and remind yourself to focus on what is best for you as a couple.

9. Don't put your life on hold. Continue living the life God granted you. Be sure to avoid wasting time worrying about tomorrow. Live one day at a time.

10. Don't feel guilty about avoiding social situations that are painful to you right now.

11. Allow yourself to grieve (you will read about this in Chapter 10).

12. Seek the support of others who have been through similar experiences. There are two sources with listings of support groups in Appendix A.

13. Accept that you are not in control.

Be sure to pray and ask for God's will about further testing or other options like Janet did. While experiencing secondary infertility she and her husband "opened three doors" so to speak and allowed God to shut them as He saw fit. She was at a point where she looked me in the face and said with all honesty that she would accept *whatever* God's plan was for her family.

This gave her and her husband forward momentum and it taught them lessons in faith. This is how she recollects that time in her life: *"After attending our infertility support group,"* Janet said. *"I learned that God did have a plan for me and he was not punishing me. During the study, we learned about dealing with the issue through surrender. I left the study with my carefully planned surrender outline: I prayed that God would bless me one of three ways. The first was to try an IVF cycle one time. Second, if that didn't work, I would proceed to adoption. Third, if it seemed clear that God wanted me to dedicate my life to raising my one and only child Jake, I would.*

So, leaving the study with my new tools, I began my plan—little did I know that God was going to test me. Two weeks after the care group ended, my IVF cycle failed. A week later my sister called to tell me that she accidentally ended up pregnant (after already having four children). I remember her crying and saying, 'Why didn't God just give you this baby?' She felt so guilty... like she took a baby that was supposed to be for me.

What came out of my mouth was this: 'that wasn't God's plan for us.' Wow! That felt so good to say (and truly believe it as well)! She got really quiet on the phone and I continued. God has a special plan for both of us that we can't see right now. I couldn't believe how calm I felt when I got off the phone with her. How very thankful I felt that Christi hosted this care group so I could learn how to listen to God and understand these things better."

Janet confides that if she had not had a care group and learned how to surrender to God, she wouldn't have reacted in such a positive way. She says she probably would have been very bitter, angry and jealous. *"There would have been a million questions such as 'Why not me God?' and 'Why her, when she already has four beautiful children?' I may have slammed a few doors, and my poor husband would have spent weeks trying to console me only to have it backfire into another pity party. But I didn't do any of those things,"* she said.

"Okay, I thought, onto my surrender plan of adoption. I went on to complete all the necessary paperwork to adopt. Through this process, I got to see how important it is to obey my husband and that the decisions he makes are from God's plan for our family. I got to hear from my social worker some of the most beautiful things my husband had said about me. It gave our marriage an even more intimate and loving relationship," Janet recalled.

Ironically, when Janet and Ed got to the point where they were ready to be introduced to birth mothers, Janet found out she was pregnant. Furthermore, two years later she and her husband went back to the same agency, spent a year going through the same proceedings, and as soon as they got to the point where they were ready to be introduced to birth mothers, she found out she was pregnant again. God really does have a great sense of humor! *"It's funny how my surrender plans weren't God's plan at all!"* Janet concluded.

"If any of you lacks wisdom, he should ask God, who gives generously to all with out finding fault, and it will be given to him." James 1:5

What to Expect From Infertility Tests

Whenever our "club" gets together and one of the ladies is going in for a test, she naturally wants to know what to expect from the rest of us. Instead of whipping out our color brochures and reading the sterile, detailed, medical terminology, we prepare her by what I call "girl talk." I have asked these wonderful friends to describe what you should expect from individual tests using this kind of terminology. We truly hope it is helpful. If you need more precise or formal written information, consult your doctor.

Before we get to the girl talk, my husband, Shawn Kari, DVM, gives a basic overview of what your husband's tests will include:

CHAPTER 9—OPENING YOUR MIND TO OTHER PLANS GOD HAS FOR YOU

Semen Analysis, Sperm Penetration Assay (Hamster Egg Penetration Test)

"Infertility generally begins with the man. Not only as the ultimate source of the problem but in testing. It is easiest and most cost effective to evaluate the man's capacity to reproduce (fertilize) and infinitely less painful. A good reproductive physical checkup is paramount. Evaluation of the prostate, presence of varicoceles and testicular anomalies are relatively easy and pain-free to perform, albeit a bit embarrassing sometimes. Additionally, a baseline blood test and tests for venereal diseases as well as certain hormone levels may also be indicated. But the "sperm count" remains the mainstay of the male reproductive workup.

The sperm count is somewhat of a misnomer. Actually **semen analysis** *is the more accurate term. A semen analysis consists of the total number of sperm per ejaculate, an evaluation of shape and morphology, and most importantly progressive motility. Sperm demonstrating a definiteness of purpose or progressive motility are needed if fertilization is to occur regardless of the overall number of sperm present. The results of the semen analysis are a reasonable assessment of whether or not a man is capable of fertilization. A sub-normal semen analysis will likely need one or two more evaluations to establish a diagnosis of male sub-infertility,"* Dr. Kari said.

He says a sperm penetration or "Hamster Egg Penetration Test" is often performed if the semen analysis is within normal limits. The ability of a man's sperm to penetrate a hamster's egg (in a petri dish) generally correlates well with how a man's sperm can penetrate human eggs. The HEPT evaluates the sperms ability to penetrate the egg once it completes its long journey. This test is generally accepted as the best test to determine the fertilizing capabilities of a man's sperm. Like any test, the HEPT is not 100% accurate. In fact, as many as 10% of men who's sperm do not pass the test impregnate their partners. Likewise, some men whose sperm perform well in the test fail to impregnate their partners.

Last, Dr. Kari says the doctor may need to take semen cultures for a variety of genital tract infections and to determine if sperm agglutination (clumping and interfering with progressive motility) is present. The doctor may also need to take X-rays or an ultrasound evaluation of the organs involved in reproduction. If a problem is identified, there may be a variety of treatments available.

Charting Your Cycle, Clomid, the Hysterosalpingogram and the Postcoital Test

Next, doctors usually sit down with both of you and report the results of your husband's tests. If further tests need to be done, or if a surgical procedure must be scheduled, you will be advised. Otherwise, if the tests are negative, your doctor will describe the course of action he has planned for you, the wife, according to your medical history.

The following account is from Charlene; she describes **Charting your Cycle**, the fertility drug "**Clomid**," the **Hysterosalpingogram** and the **Postcoital Test**.

*"Once the doctor determined it would be safe to conceive, I was taught how to **chart my cycles**. This method of family planning involves charting the basil body temperature by using a thermometer every morning. When my temperature spiked, it was supposed to be the optimal baby-making time and my husband was 'on duty.'*

Now let me explain something. First of all, I wouldn't even remember to get up in the morning if my paycheck didn't depend on it. Now I was expected to wake up at the same time every day and immediately remember to stick a thermometer in my mouth before I got up to use the restroom or anything. Second, men only think about sex all the time. They don't really want sex all the time—trust me. After a couple of months of sex-on-demand I thought he was going to run screaming from the house every time I told him my temperature had spiked.

*When that didn't work after a couple of months, I started taking a low-dose fertility drug called **Clomid** in hopes it would increase the number of eggs my ovaries popped out each month.*

The doctor mentioned there might be some minor side effects. Let me tell you—the hormonal havoc these fertility chemicals wreak on the body makes PMS look like a stroll on the beach. If I wasn't curled in a ball sobbing on the couch, I was doing a pretty convincing impression of Attila the Hun.

Month after month I continued to bleed and sank deeper and deeper into a fit of depression (which I'm sure doesn't help the conception rate). The only thing that I think saved my sanity was joining an infertility support Bible study through my church. When that ended, my family was begging me to find another source of support.

CHAPTER 9—OPENING YOUR MIND TO OTHER PLANS GOD HAS FOR YOU

Next, I went through another regimen of tests. The worst one was the **Hysterosalpingogram**. *(I call it the Hysterical Ping-o-Gram). To say this test won't hurt is like saying being dragged behind a Mack Truck won't give you road rash."*

Charlene says in simple terms, this test is an X-ray of the fallopian tubes. You are required to lie down on the X-ray table in nothing but a hospital gown. The technician takes some preliminary X-rays of the pelvic area. Then, he or she inserts into your vagina a long, plastic tube connected to a syringe filled with dye. Charlene said, *"It wasn't so bad until she started injecting the dye – it felt like liquid fire. I laid on the table and cried as the technician took more X-rays while the dye traveled into my body, up my fallopian tubes and out again. The idea was to document any blockages there may be in the fallopian tubes or corresponding body parts. All of the pain was for nothing. There were no blockages and the doctor couldn't see anything else wrong with my 'equipment.'*

After the Hysterical Ping-o-Gram was negative and my husband's sperm count and motility tested normal, we did a **postcoital test**. *This test is exactly what it sounds like. My husband and I had to have sex, then immediately go into the doctor's office so they could retrieve a sample out of me. It was one of the most embarrassing things I've ever done. On the other hand, it turned out to be the most important because we finally determined what was wrong!*

We learned my body was rejecting the sperm. There was nothing wrong with either of us individually, but together, we were like rain on a campfire. I just extinguished anything he put in there," Charlene concluded.

Pergonal, Metrodin, Lupron and Synarel Fertility Drugs

In addition to Clomid, **Pergonal** and **Metrodin** are used to stimulate ovulation. As I understand, they are injected, meaning you will be receiving a shot daily (probably from your husband), several office visits are required, each cycle of shots are rather expensive, and there are side effects.

Lupron and **Synarel**—Because I have a great fear of needles, I chose to take the nasal spray, Synarel, over the injector, Lupron. Both are designed to suppress the production of estrogen. My doctor's goal was to shrink the amount of endometriosis I was experiencing, so he basically used chemicals to "put me into menopause" for six months. I was so miserable I only made it five months.

From that experience I have this advice to pass on: The next time you are around an older woman who is going through "the change," have pity on her my friends. The hot flashes and night sweats are horrible. You don't just feel warm, you feel like you are burning inside. In addition, the crankiness, mood swings and instability actually left me begging my doctor for a hysterectomy.

Endometrial Biopsy and Laparoscopy

I agree with Charlene that the postcoital test was rather embarrassing. I also agree that the hysterosalpingogram was a bit painful, but the test I didn't tolerate well was the **Endometrial Biopsy**. You will be advised to have someone available to drive you home after this test and your doctor will recommend that you take some form of pain medication 30 minutes before the procedure.

Once you are placed in the stirrups, the doctor will place a biopsy needle in your vagina. It will puncture your uterus and pull out a piece to be analyzed. Your muscles will automatically contract leaving you extremely sore for about an hour. If you forget to take the pain relief beforehand, prepare for a very uncomfortable ride home.

If you have undergone all of these tests, the next step is usually a **Laparoscopy.** This is an outpatient surgery, so be prepared to have someone drive you home, and plan on about two days to a week to fully recuperate depending on your level of pain tolerance.

Once in the hospital, you will receive an IV and then general anesthesia. The surgeon will make a small incision below your belly button and one a few inches lower. He or she will fill your abdomen with gas and then check your reproductive organs for endometriosis, scar tissue, cysts, etc. A laser will be used to clean out your fallopian tubes if necessary. Normally, it only takes 2-3 hours for you to recover and unless you have a bad reaction to the anesthesia, the doctor will allow you to go home once you prove that you are able to urinate.

You will be a little tender in the abdominal area, however I didn't think the pain was bad at all. The discomfort I felt was the gas leaving my body through the shoulder blades for two to three days.

Once you've undergone the laparoscopy, your doctor will probably give you the green light to act like bunnies in the bedroom, because the next three months are an exceptionally good time for conception.

CHAPTER 9—OPENING YOUR MIND TO OTHER PLANS
GOD HAS FOR YOU

What to Expect from Advanced Procedures

If all of your tests return negative, or if the medical community discloses problems that can only be corrected through advanced techniques, you will probably be advised to sit down with your husband and contemplate Artificial Insemination (AI), Intra-Uterine Insemination (IUI), In Vitro Fertilization (IVF), Gamete Intra-Fallopian Transfer (GIFT), Zygote Intra-Fallopian Transfer (ZIFT), or any other procedure your specialist may have in mind. In my opinion, these procedures require more commitment, in addition to money and time, plus your emotions will be more intense. On the flip side, these procedures often yield great results!

Intra-Uterine Insemination and Artificial Insemination

Charlene describes **Intra-Uterine Insemination**. (By the way, the difference between **Artificial Insemination** and IUI is this: with AI, the catheter inserts the husband's sperm just outside the cervix, whereas with IUI, the sperm is placed directly into the uterus.) *"Because my body was rejecting my husband's sperm, my doctor suggested we try a procedure called Intra-Uterine Insemination. The idea was to get the sperm higher into my body, past the point where I was killing all of them off. After more than two years of tests, temperature taking, pills and praying, I was willing to try one more thing...but I wasn't going to hold my breath.*

I continued to take the Clomid, chart my temperature, and go to the hospital every day right around the peak of my cycle for an internal ultrasound. On February 5, 2000, my temperature spiked and the ultrasound showed an egg in my fallopian tube. My husband was sent into a private room with a cup. He was given no magazines, no videos, or other aides and he was very nervous and embarrassed. He declined my offer to come in with him, strip naked and do the hula. Let's just say it was a good thing the doctor was after quality and not quantity. His nerves really reduced the volume.

His sperm was given to a lab technician who put them into a machine that I thought of as a sperm-merry-go-round. It 'washed' the sperm by spinning it in a machine, weeding out all the weak sperm and leaving the strong swimmers. After that was done, I went into a room with a gown on. The nurse had a syringe of his sperm connected to a plastic tube that immediately reminded me of the Hysterical-Ping-o-Gram. She assured me it wouldn't hurt... and it didn't. I didn't even feel her insert the tube and gently release the sperm into the upper part of my pelvic area.

Five minutes later I was dressed, out the door, and on my way to work. For the next two weeks I was a nervous wreck. I noticed every little twitch in my body wondering if it was a sign of pregnancy or an oncoming period. A week after the procedure I went out of state for a writer's conference. I had a hard time concentrating during what should have been a restful time of creative exploration because I started having cramps. I began to get depressed until I realized that although I had cramps, I wasn't bleeding.

Finally, about 15 days after the procedure, I couldn't take it any more. I went to the store and bought a pregnancy test. It was positive. I was going to be a mom. I had heard of women trying insemination and in-vitro fertilization for years before they conceived. I couldn't believe it only took one time and thanked God over and over (and to this day) that it only took once for us.

I wondered why we couldn't have done the IUI sooner, but I know why now. The prolonged waiting and the profuse wanting made the success that much sweeter – her name is Kayla Irene Engeron and she means the world to us."

In Vitro Fertilization, Gamete Intra-Fallopian Transfer and Zygote Intra-Fallopian Transfer

Janet describes what to expect from **IVF, GIFT and ZIFT:** *"Before attempting any of these procedures, you definitely want to clear your calendars since it really is a three-month process from start to finish. You want the least amount of stress as possible!! There are really five stages that you will go through during these types of procedures.*

The First Procedure is Considered the Preliminary Stage

This is when there will be many tests done. It will take a lot of coordinating and timing between your schedule, your husband's calendar, the reproductive endocrinologist (RE), the laboratory that draws your blood, and any other commitments you my have. There will be lots of paperwork to complete such as consent forms, insurance forms (if it is covered) and maybe

CHAPTER 9—OPENING YOUR MIND TO OTHER PLANS
GOD HAS FOR YOU

even financial agreements. You will meet with your RE doctor to go over all the 'what if's,' followed by a semen screening, infectious disease screening and various other blood tests

At times it will seem very overwhelming, but I suggest that you make a chart and list the needed tests and paperwork. This will help you remain organized. I also recommend that you read through all the information given to you. The more knowledge you arm yourself with, the easier it is to make informative decisions and ask the appropriate questions.

The Secondary Stage is Considered the Pituitary Desensitization

When your cycle begins, you will go to your RE's office to begin the shots needed for this stage. You and your husband will be shown how to draw up the meds from the vial and into the syringe. Then you will be instructed on how to give subcutaneous injections (meaning just below the skin). The nurse will have you practice first on an orange and then as your husband perfects the orange and his confidence builds, he will then perform his first injection. Since it is a subcutaneous injection, it really is fairly easy and not too painful. It is usually administered in the upper thigh. However, the drug (usually Lupron) does burn as it enters the system, but with a little rubbing at the site from hubby, it passes.

This phase usually lasts about 10 days. You may experience hot flashes, weight gain, crankiness and irritability, as well as bruising on the thighs. You may also have to take various other meds such as baby aspirin or other oral medication at this time.

The Third Stage is Called the "Controlled Ovarian Hyperstimulation"

In my opinion, this stage is the hardest physically. You will continue your Lupron injections along with another set of injections. The drug you will begin helps with the development of eggs (Oocytes). There are various types and names for the drug used. Depending on the brand name used for your stimulation drug, it will either be injected subcutaneous or may need to be injected intramuscularly. In the latter case, you will be instructed on how to do an intra muscular injection, which usually is done in the buttocks (so, be extra nice to your husband during this time period!).

You then will be seen in the office every two to three days. They will draw your blood to test for hormone levels and they will do a vaginal ultrasound to *determine the number of eggs you are producing. At this point, the mental and physical part of this cycle will start to wear on you. There are so many shots to take and doctor's appointments to schedule. Physically you will be dealing with bloating, ovary tenderness, raging hormones, fatigue, and restlessness. Again this stage does end usually between 10-16 days depending on the individual.*

The Fourth Stage is Called the Egg (Oocyte) Retrieval

At this point, the eggs (oocytes) have been fully matured. You will be given an HCG shot intramuscularly at the re's office and sent home. What this shot does is trigger ovulation to occur in approximately 42-48 hours. After the needed amount of time passes, the eggs will be retrieved by transvaginal aspiration.

This procedure is done as an outpatient procedure. You will be put under light sedation and vaginally the doctor will go in to remove the eggs via a long needle with a tube like hose. After waking up, you may feel groggy or lightheaded. You may feel some tenderness in the ovary area, but a little painkiller should help. You will be sent home and allowed to do only light activities.

The Fifth Stage is Called the Post-Transfer Phase

During this phase many scenarios come into play. The main purpose of this stage is that the egg/sperm are united. The most popular ways are as follows:

IVF: *This is where the egg and sperm are put into a petri dish and fertilized to become an embryo. They are then placed back into the upper most part of the cervix.*
GIFT: *This is where the egg and sperm are handled separately and placed back into the upper fallopian tubes via laparoscopy.*
ZIFT: *This is where the egg and sperm are put into a petri dish and fertilized to become an embryo. Then the embryo is placed in the fallopian tubes via laparoscopy.*

The goal is to produce life—an embryo. I will go into more detail in regards to the actual process of an IVF procedure at this time. At this point,

CHAPTER 9—OPENING YOUR MIND TO OTHER PLANS GOD HAS FOR YOU

they will monitor the embryos and usually 48 hours later, if the embryos make it, they will call you to come in for the transfer. This is a very exciting and very scary time.

Once you arrive, they will take you into a treatment room. You will undress from the waist down. The doctor will come in with a tube (your embryos) and place the tube into the vagina with the number of embryos you and your doctor have discussed. It is not too painful; it will be similar to what you would feel during an annual pap smear. The doctor will have you lay there for 45 minutes. It is a long time and many thoughts go through your mind: Will I become a mother? Will I be a mother of twins? Do I feel them attaching to the uterine wall? Or, are they lost?

Then the doctor will have you go home and lay down for the next 12-24 hours. Each doctor will have his own protocol as to the amount of activity, diet and exercise you can do during this time period. He will then have you begin taking Progesterone. This can be taken vaginally as a suppository or it may have to be injected intramuscularly. This will be taken until your pregnancy is confirmed. Then comes the long and final wait. It usually is about a 10-12-day wait after which you will go in for a pregnancy test."

Janet adds that during her IVF Cycle she relied on two positive outlooks: 1) That she was physically and financially able to take advantage of this option, and 2) That she and her husband made the decision to do it together.

She concludes, *"Think of it this way. I told myself that every morning when I got up, I was an IVF patient while taking my shots. After the shots were done, I became my normal self for the rest of the day. I didn't let that IVF patient follow me around for the rest of the day. There was always the next day to play patient."*

Considering Adoption

The "picture" of adoption has changed drastically over the years. Back in the 50's and 60's, unwed mothers were social outcasts. Typically they were shunned by their families and forced to hide somewhere until their babies were born. Many of them weren't even allowed to see their newborns before they were placed in the arms of awaiting adoptive parents. That's why you continue to see so many women searching for the children they have agonized over all these years.

Even now, considering adoption is a big decision. What is bigger?—The number of children in the world who need homes. When contemplating

adoption, I suggest you address these five questions as a couple:
1. Will you concentrate on domestic or international adoption?
2. Do you intend to go through your county, an attorney-based organization, or an agency?
3. Do you prefer a newborn, toddler, older child, or a special needs child?
4. Are you comfortable with an open, semi-open or closed adoption?
5. Would you prefer to give birth to your adopted child? (*See Giving Birth to Your Adopted Child –Embryo Adoptions.*)

The answers to these questions will help you narrow down which organizations will fit your needs. Next, go on a fact-finding tour of each organization you are interested in. Attend their orientations and get answers to your questions until one of them "clicks" with you. You'll know it, or you'll walk away knowing this option isn't for you.

From what I have seen and experienced first hand, the adoption process takes about a year and can take up to five years (once again, this depends on the type of adoption you choose). Every adoption experience is different and every organization, county, and country has different specifications and requisites.

My Experience—Semi-Open Christian Adoption Through an Agency

My personal experience was with Bethany Christian Services (a nationwide agency that can be reached at 1-800-BETHANY or www.bethany.org). After attending their orientation, we completed a preliminary application. Once we were accepted, the formal application process included a thick packet of paperwork to complete. It took us three months to return the following (things have changed and this packet may be quite different now, however, I want to convey to you that a lot of paperwork is normally required with any adoption process):

1. Formal application, family histories, questionnaires, profiles and autobiographies
2. Doctor's records
3. Employment verification
4. Affidavit of health insurance
5. Fingerprint cards and child abuse index
6. DMV verification
7. Proof of First Aid/CPR class attendance
8. Copies of tax returns

CHAPTER 9—OPENING YOUR MIND TO OTHER PLANS GOD HAS FOR YOU

9. Copies of birth certificates, marriage certificates, divorce decrees

To be perfectly honest, I was astonished at this list. In my naïve mind, I thought these people would welcome us in and thank us for considering adoption. I found myself irritated that pregnant 12-year-olds don't have to complete a packet like this. On the other hand, I understand that agencies feel responsible for the children they are placing in homes, thus the need for a thorough background check is needed.

Once we cleared this hurdle, Bethany arranged four counseling sessions that were very helpful. I was dealing with a lot of fear at the time. I kept telling my counselor, *"I can't handle the thought of a knock on my door from a mother wanting her baby back!"* She helped me deal with those anxieties. We also discussed adoption-related issues that will arise, as well as handling situations in the future such as when my children say, *"I don't have to obey you – you're not my real mom!"*

Next, we sat down with the director to specify what traits we hoped to be matched up with including physical looks of the birth parents and nationalities that mixed with ours. For example, my father-in-law was a prisoner of war for eight years in Vietnam. We called him and asked how he would feel if our adopted child looked Asian. His answer was affirmative – *"No problem,"* he said. It was very important to us that our child have loving relationships with grandparents, as well as aunts and uncles, so making phone calls to our family helped narrow down our "wish list."

We also had to indicate what health issues we thought we could handle such as "drug babies," babies born with a clubfoot, heart murmur, etc. This was very difficult for me because I felt like I was "ordering" a baby like I order a meal in a restaurant: *I'd like a cute little girl, blond hair, brown eyes, with great sports abilities, hold the attitude, and extra sweetness on the side please.* In actuality, God had predetermined what children would be placed in our home and this stage of the process was intended to link us to the birth mothers who were carrying those children.

Likewise, it was necessary to determine how much, if any, contact we would accept with the birth parents. This is done so that a birth mother's "wish list" could be matched with ours. For example, if we preferred a closed adoption, our "profile" would not be shown to a birth mother who preferred a continued relationship.

In our situation, our profile was shown to birth mothers until one selected us to parent her child (sometimes birth fathers are involved too). The agency determined if we would meet each other before or after the baby's birth according to the pre-established wishes of both parties involved. In case you are interested, both of our adoptions totaled $15,000 in 1999.

We chose **semi-open adoptions** meaning we met the birth parents, however, no last names or hometowns were divulged and future contact would only be accepted if agreed upon by both parties. I will continue to send letters and pictures of my children to their birth parents until they are 18 years of age (our agency forwards the mail in envelopes bearing their return address, not ours).

Last, at some point you and your spouse must determine how you will make your child(ren) aware of their adoption. My husband and I have chosen to make our children aware from the beginning. We believe that when you keep secrets, or withhold such valuable information, or you lie to your children, their resulting rebellion will be immense. We believe they will have a solid foundation in their young lives this way and we feel no threat because *we* are their parents.

Jeannine's Experience–Open, Private, Attorney-Based Adoption

Many times adoption isn't our idea, it's God's. After several years of marriage without the use of birth control, Russell and Jeannine knew something was wrong, however, they chose not to seek medical help. After 11 years they knew they would either remain a family of two or they would have to visit the idea of adoption.

"Sometimes you can feel God acting in your life and you just know he's trying to show you the way. In early 2001 we began our first step down the path that God planned for us so many years earlier. My wife, Jeannine, met a three-year-old boy who was being cared for by his grandparents and she learned that they were looking for a family to take him in. After a heartfelt discussion, we decided to pursue the possibility of adopting him. After three months of trying, we were to be disappointed once again. It turned out that the grandparents had only temporary custody, and they weren't ready to give him up after all.

September would hold the blessing we were waiting for. The mother of a close friend called one day to tell us she met a 17-year-old girl who was eight months pregnant and wanted a loving home for her baby. We were thrilled, and agreed to meet her that weekend. We knew right away that she was a sweetheart, and within the hour she decided that we were the perfect choice. We asked a lot of questions and so did she. We wanted to know about drug abuse, and if there was any chance of her changing her mind. We left tearfully hugging one another, as everyone's prayers had just been answered. Now it was time to get to work. We had a baby to adopt.

After Bryson's birth, (in October of 2001), we felt an obligation to provide closure for his birthmother and her family. We didn't feel right about walking away with this beautiful child and leaving them with nothing. Our family and friends cautioned us about keeping them out of the picture, but our hearts told us otherwise. We invited them to become an extended part of our family so that they too could share in Bryson's life. Our philosophy is that the more people he has in his life to love him, the better," explained Russell.

Once the Kingstons decided to adopt Bryson, they located an attorney, a social worker through the county, and then a service provider (an agency) to provide for the birth mother's rights, (she had rights for 90 days after Bryson's birth). After the birth mother released her rights and the required paperwork was completed, it was 10 months later when the family went to court to finalize the adoption.

Russell adds the following about **open adoption**: *"Bryson's birthmother kept her distance at first, probably to protect herself emotionally. We left it up to her to decide how involved she wanted to be. In a short time, she has become like a daughter to us, and will hopefully remain an important part in all our lives. This has been our journey thus far. A man and wife tormented by the intricacies of conception are blessed in ways they never imagined. In the end two hearts become three, and the dream continues..."*

Michelle's Experience—Closed, Agency-Based International Adoption

Michelle and her husband, Shawn, had three biological children when they chose to adopt siblings from Russia. Because they chose international adoption through Nightlight Christian Adoptions in California (www.nightlight.org), their adoption was considered **closed** (since there was no chance of future contact with the birth parents).

Normally, there are two required trips to the country of origin: one, to visit or choose the child, and the second, to complete the legalities and take the child home. Some couples choose the children they adopt before they go abroad. Others visit orphanages or adoption agencies within the country they are interested in and choose their adopted child(ren) in person.

Michelle was looking for "open doors" from God as to who would be her children. How does God show us His plans for us? We've talked about some ways: through prayer, scripture, through what godly people in your life say or do, and through circumstances. So, she went to Nightlight's office to look through books of children waiting for homes and no "doors opened" for her.

She decided to make another visit and take her five-year-old daughter because she knew an innocent child would not be slanted in her choices. When they were looking through the pictures of children at the agency, she saw a page with a brother and sister on it whom she hadn't seen before. Upon inquiry, her social worker said their profile had just been inserted, so Michelle and her daughter, Alli, decided to watch a video profile. In the video, the Russian girl said that she liked dollies and Alli turned to Michelle and said, "*I have dollies.*" The girl proceeded to say that she liked Barbie dolls, and Alli turned to Michelle and said, "*I have lots of Barbies.*"

Looking back, Michelle said she still needed more evidence from God, so she showed Alli a pair of really cute sisters, and Alli replied to her mother, "*No, that was my brother and sister!*" Still, Michelle admits she wasn't paying attention to the great big door (and window) God had opened, so on the way home, she decided that if the Russian girl's name was said, she'd know it was God's will to adopt this pair. She listened to talk radio—no mention of the name "Katia." Later, she called her friend, Jan, and told her about the Russian siblings, and Jan said, "*Oh, I wonder if that is the same Katia my daughter, Emily, loved so much while in the orphanage. Does she have a brother named Alosha?*" Michelle replied "yes," and realized immediately she had her answer all along!

International adoptions require paperwork through an agency or attorney, two trips to the country of origin and they can cost up to $30,000. Try not to let that figure discourage you; there is literature available (see Appendix A) that will assist you with creative financing ideas and facts about tax advantages.

Julie's Experience—Fos-Dopt Through the County

Julie and her husband, Sam, were devastated when a child they intended to adopt through a private establishment was returned to her birth mother. "*We were heart broken to lose Annie, but I have faith that God had a different plan for her life,*" Julie confided. After raising Annie from nine months to the age of two, Julie knew she wanted to try adoption again.

"*I started looking into agency and lawyer-based adoptions and was then *told about adoption through the county, so I looked into it. It didn't take long and we were paired up with a baby girl. After she was born, it was difficult for my husband to fully give Tessa his heart, because her birth father had to be located to relinquish his rights. We didn't finalize the adoption for a year and a half. Once that took place, Sam's fears were removed and he was able to relax and enjoy her even more,"* Julie explained.

Typically counties use the Fos-dopt Program, meaning you foster the child you intend to adopt until the parents' rights are relinquished and the adoption is finalized in court. Once again, every adoption is different, so you may wait up to five years to go through the process. In the meantime, you are required to complete paperwork and attend training seminars. Often an adoption through the county is only $500.00 (depending on your location and the situation of the child).

If you are interested in adopting through your county, start out by contacting your County's Children's Services Office. The easiest way to do this is to look under the "government" pages in the front of your phone book, titled "Government Offices, County." Next, look under the Department of Children's Services or the Child Welfare Services. This should include Foster Care, Fos-Dopt, and Adoption services.

The Difference Between Relinquishing and Releasing Birth Parents' Rights

When you adopt within the United States, I personally condone agency adoptions over lawyer-based or facilitator adoptions because the birth mother (or birth parents) undergo counseling sessions to make them fully aware of their rights and their decision. As I understand, the birth parents cannot reverse their rights to their child later citing coercion.

Because of this knowledge on the birth parents' behalf, in most agencies, the birth mother is only given 24 hours to change her mind after she gives birth. When that period is up, both birth parents sign a paper **relinquishing** their rights to their child *forever*. When our two adoptions fell through, it was because during the 24 hour-period family, friends, and even hospital staff besieged the birth mothers with guilt.

On the other hand, with lawyer-based and facilitator adoptions, if they do not pair up with an agency, there is no counseling for the birth parents therefore, when they sign over their rights it is a **release** for six months or so.

These are the failed adoptions they make movies out of, however, I don't want to sound critical because I know their success rates are high too. The point is, choose your agency, lawyer or facilitator very carefully. If you choose a facilitator from the Internet, be especially careful and take the time to look into their history and ratings with the Better Business Bureau or consumer protection agencies beforehand.

Giving Birth to Your Adopted Child (Embryo Adoptions)

According to a Nightlight Christian Adoptions brochure, *"Embryos preserved in frozen storage offer great hope for life and for families facing fertility challenges. When a family has been successful in having a child through IVF, embryos are often cryo-preserved, resulting in the questions of what to do with them. These frozen embryos can be the hope of a child for an infertile couple. Embryo adoption shares this wonderful hope with others.*

In 1997, Nightlight began the Snowflakes Frozen Embryo Adoption Program, which is helping some of the more than 400,000 frozen embryos realize their ultimate purpose – life – while sharing the hope of a child with an infertile couple. In addition to your physician, you need to trust the people you choose to help you in these important decisions."

The best way to learn about this option is to inquire about the "Snowflakes Embryo Adoption Program" through the Nightlight website at www.nightlight.org or contact an agency that provides this service in your area.

Last, I want to add that what tickles me about adoption is watching God's sense of humor. It never ceases to amaze me how our two children look like siblings, although they have different birth parents. Adopted children often share their adoptive parents' characteristics therefore, comments such as *"she's got your eyes,"* and *"Oh, it looks like he's got his daddy's height,"* are common. Adopted children also pick up their parents' mannerisms. I giggle under my breath every time someone tells me, *"Your son asks just like your husband!"*

"Religion that God our Father accepts as pure and faultless is this: to look after orphans and widows in their distress and to keep oneself from being polluted by the world." **James 1:27**

CHAPTER 9—OPENING YOUR MIND TO OTHER PLANS
GOD HAS FOR YOU

What to Consider Before You Adopt

Because you are making a life altering, "forever" decision, it is important that you and your husband talk to adoptive parents, read books, and research this subject as best as possible before you take action.

In my biased opinion, adoption is an awesome privilege. I'll never, ever forget how I felt the day the agency representatives placed our baby daughter in my arms. I was in love with her instantly. This is probably because I had been praying about this child, her birth parents and even her life in utero for a year. As we placed our bundle of joy in the car that day, I looked back at the agency thinking, *are they really going to let us take this little miracle home?*

Just because God selected me to be the mother of Alexis doesn't mean I'm a perfect parent. I make all the usual mistakes others make. In fact, rearing children is much more difficult than I ever imagined. I thought I would naturally know how to handle situations— not true! I watch others, I read articles and books and frankly, I experiment to see what works and doesn't work.

I also expected to bond as easily and naturally with my son, Jesse, as I did with my daughter. The problem was at one-week-old he cried one evening for nine straight hours. I took him to the doctor and they diagnosed colic. This is a condition where the doctors can't explain why the baby's digestive system causes them great pain. The gas and pressure causes them to emit a piercing scream and uncontrollable crying for long periods of time.

Because Jesse cried night and day for the next eight, long months, I couldn't bond with him. He didn't want to be rocked, sang to or read to. None of my efforts to be a loving, gentle, problem-fixing mother worked. I had to constantly remind myself of the 10 years of waiting and begging the Lord for this child. I had to make a concerted effort to love him and finally, after four years the love came naturally.

I'm telling you this so you will be prepared, not fearful. Adopted children aren't perfect; they do not grow into appreciative, little people thanking you and respecting you because you gave them a home. They are innocent, little souls gifted to you to nurture and help mold into the people God created them to be.

If you're still wrestling with the question, *"Can I love another person's child?"* Barbara has great advice to share. She says, *"If you are wondering whether you have the capability to love a child not born to you, ask yourself this question: 'Do you want to be parents?' There is a difference between being a parent and wanting a child simply to make sure the family name is carried on, or wanting a 'little me.' A parent is someone who takes on the responsibility of raising and caring for a child in love, regardless of specific traits or 'genes.' It's unconditional love, plain and simple. Parents desire to see their child become all that God wants him or her to be, and they willingly make sacrifices to ensure the best possible outcome.*

For me, adoption has been an awesome privilege. The hole that was in my life for many years has been filled to overflowing. I could never have imagined the outpouring of love that I now feel for our child. All of the pain and sorrow that I felt for so long has evaporated. I am having the experiences that I longed for in years past. God has given me my heart's desire, although not in the way I had always planned for it to happen. I have come to realize that adoption is not settling for second best, it is just another path to the goal of parenthood," [8]

Once people find out my children are adopted, so many of them say, *"I've always wanted to adopt."* It's an interesting statement, because I wonder, *Well, then what's stopping you?* Ninety percent of the time their excuse is that it's too expensive. I admit that you will spend between $15,000 –30,000 per adoption depending on whether you adopt domestically or internationally.

We knew we wanted to adopt domestically and the two biggest factors that helped us narrow down an agency were 1) we preferred a Christian organization, and 2) we wanted a non-profit organization. I didn't want to feel like I was "buying" a baby. Instead, our not-for-profit agency's fee was based upon a percentage of our income and the director sat down and considered our bills when we established the bottom line. What impressed me the most is that with both adoptions, *I called them after a week* of having our child in the home asking when they wanted payment.

I want to add one last thing about the financial aspects of adoption. Most people I know will go to a car dealer and sign on the bottom line promising to make monthly payments so that they can leave the lot driving a nice, shiny, new $20-30,000 car, van, truck or SUV. I get a little defensive when they try to tell me about their new car in the same breath as, *"Adoption is too expensive."* We didn't have that kind of money in our savings account, so our bank gave us both of our adoption loans.

Whatever you decide, make sure it's best for your family. Try not to let others influence your decision too much. If adoption doesn't feel right and you decide to remain a complete family of two, three or four… move on with your lives (the next chapter tells you how) knowing that you have made an intelligent, thoughtful, honest decision to the best of your abilities.

CHAPTER 9—OPENING YOUR MIND TO OTHER PLANS GOD HAS FOR YOU

Legacy of An Adopted Child

Once there were two women
Who never knew each other.
One you do not remember,
The other you call mother.

Two different lives
Shaped to make yours one.
One became your guiding star,
The other became your sun.

The first gave you life
And the second taught you to live in it.
The first gave you a need for love
And the second was there to give it.
One gave you a nationality,
The other gave you a name.
One gave you the seed of talent,
The other gave you an aim.

One gave you emotions,
The other calmed your fears.
One saw your first sweet smile,
The other dried your tears.

One gave you up,
It was all that she could do.
The other prayed for a child
And God lead her straight to you.

And now you ask me
Through your tears,
The age-old question
Through the years:

Heredity or environment,
Which are you the product of?
Neither, my darling, neither,
Just two kinds of LOVE!

Author Unknown

Considering Foster Care

If you determine that you are unable to conceive a child and you are not quite sure about adoption, consider foster care. I would start out by contacting your county office. Look in your phone book (see instructions in the previous section for their address and phone number) or call local agencies and inquire about foster care.

Once you call, they will inform you of your county's requirements and also the training you will need to go through. Here is what a woman named Janet says about her experience: "*My husband and I never thought that three years ago we would be as happy and fulfilled as we are right now. In the spring of 1992, I received a phone call informing us that our chances of having children were next to impossible due to a male infertility problem. This news came as a big shock, especially after trying to have a child for two years.*

At that point, I collected as much information as I could find on alternative ways of having a baby, including Artificial Insemination and adoption. We were really taken aback when we discovered how much these options cost and that there was really no guarantee with any of them. We prayed that the Lord would show us the right thing to do and that He would open doors for us.

We waited and waited, but every door remained closed. I think the most difficult thing we had to deal with was watching our friends starting their families and realizing that we had nothing in common with them anymore. We wanted to fit in, but without children, we didn't feel as if we did.

We have now accepted the fact that we will not be able to bear children unless the Lord performs a miracle in our lives. But along the way we have learned a very important lesson: we can experience some of the same satisfaction in having children in our lives in a very special way. The way I am referring to is through foster parenting.

In the Lord's own special way, He has opened doors like never before.

CHAPTER 9—OPENING YOUR MIND TO OTHER PLANS GOD HAS FOR YOU

Just four months ago, we heard about the many opportunities in our community to become foster parents. We decided to collect information on this option and pray about it, as we had done with all the other options we had considered.

Since then, things have happened fast! We are now foster parents to a special, nine-year-old boy. We never thought fostering would be as fulfilling as it has turned out to be. Sure, there are rough times, but the good definitely outweighs the bad.

There are so many children who have been abused physically, emotionally, or sexually by their dysfunctional families. These children NEED love, attention, security, and someone to hold them when it hurts deep inside. We give all this and more to our foster child, and he gives much more back to us.

It is as if he is ours—'on loan' from the Lord—to comfort and mend the damage that has been done to him in the past. When our job is done, our door is always open for another child in need of our love, support, and direction.

Fostering may not be for everyone, but my husband and I think of foster parenting as our ministry. After all, Jesus said, 'I was hungry and you gave me something to eat, I was thirsty and you gave me something to drink, I was a stranger and you invited me in, I needed clothes and you clothed me, I was sick and you looked after me... I tell you the truth, whatever you did for one of the least of these brothers of mine, you did for me' (Matthew 25:35-40). My husband and I know that being foster parents will bring blessings into our lives. It already has."[9]

I have so much respect and admiration for people chosen by God to provide solid, loving, Christ-centered homes to neglected and abused children. It's not everyone's calling, although I believe it is one of the higher callings in life.

"Therefore anyone who humbles himself as this little child, is the greatest in the kingdom of heaven. And any of you who welcomes a little child like this because you are mine, is welcoming me and caring for me." Matthew 18:4-5 (NLT)

Chapter Ten–Opening Your Eyes to Abundant Blessings

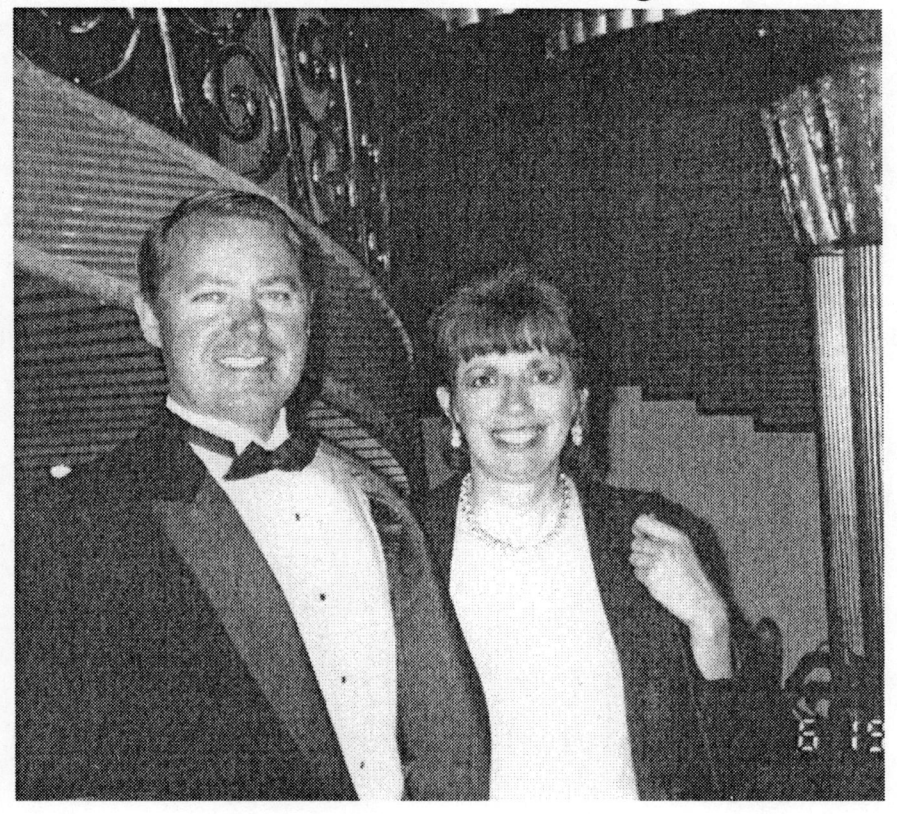

Karen and Derrick

-Grieving is a Process
    The Stages of Grief
-Blessing You is God's Gift!
    Blessings Through Spiritual Gifts
    Considering Your Spouse's Feelings
    Blessed by Marriage
    How to Strengthen a Damaged Marriage
-Moving on as a Complete Family

Chapter Ten–Opening Your Eyes to Abundant Blessings

1. Do you feel God is blessing you when it comes to infertility? Yes or No? Please explain how:

_____

_____

_____

2. Take a minute and look at your life. Is God answering other prayers in your life? Yes or No? Is He blessing you in other areas? Yes or No? Please explain both answers:

_____

_____

_____

3. Do you and your husband communicate well about the feelings you have experienced during this trial? Yes or No? How do you best express yourselves?

_____

_____

_____

4. Do you ever find yourself "attacking" your husband with blame, anger or harsh words? Yes or No? If yes, have you apologized and asked for forgiveness? Yes or No? ***Do it now!***

5. Has sex become less intimate since it is now being scheduled? Yes or No? If yes, are you doing anything to remedy this problem? Yes or No? If yes, what:

_____

_____

_____

6. Are you committed enough to your marriage, to put testing aside for a while to work on the foundation of your commitment if it comes to that? Yes or No? Are you committed enough to remain with your spouse if you find out he is sterile? Yes or No?

7. If you and your mate have decided to stop testing and continue life as a complete family, are you starting to experience peace and joy again? Yes or No? Do you feel like you're regaining balance in your life? Yes or No? List some goals or aspirations you "put on hold" during the infertility journey:

_____

_____

_____

8. Do you know what "spiritual gifts" are? Yes or No? If you do, please list your top three:
    1._____
    2._____
    3._____

9. Now list your husband's top three if you know what they are:
    1._____
    2._____
    3._____

CHAPTER 10—OPENING YOUR EYES TO ABUNDANT BLESSINGS

10. Can you think of ways you can utilize your "gifts" or fulfill some of your goals while living as a complete family of two? Please list them:

_____

_____

_____

Recommended Reading:

Psalm 103:1-16, 145:14-20
Romans 12:1-20
Colossians 3:5-12
1 Timothy 4:14-16
1 Peter 4:10-11

Matthew 6:25-34
Ephesians 2:10, 5:25-33
1 Thessalonians 5:18
James 1:19-25

Look up these verses and fill in the blanks:

1 Corinthians 12:4-11: *"There are different kinds of _____, but the same Spirit. There are different kinds of service, but the same Lord. There are different kinds of working, but the same God works all of them in all men. Now to each one the manifestation of the Spirit is given for the common good. To one there is given through the Spirit the message of wisdom, to another the message of knowledge by means of the same Spirit, to another faith by the same Spirit, to another gifts of healing by that one Spirit, to another miraculous powers, to another prophecy, to another distinguishing between spirits, to another speaking in different kinds of tongues, and to still another the interpretation of tongues. All these are the work of one and the same Spirit, and he gives them to each one, just as he _____."*

Matthew 6:34: *"Therefore do not worry about _____, for tomorrow will worry about itself. Each day has enough trouble of its own."*

"Why Won't You Bless Me God?"
Answer #9—A barren womb opens your eyes to
blessings all around you, especially
your husband and your marriage.

Chapter 10—Karen's Story

I think Derrick and I were married for almost two years before we realized there might be a problem with procreation. Before our marriage I had experienced several 'female' problems, and at the age of 28 I had emergency surgery to remove a large cyst on my left ovary and several small cysts on my right ovary. My doctor started me on birth control pills and assured me I would be able to bear children at a later date.

We married in 1989 and spent the first six months apart. Unfortunately, that was the 'picture' of our marriage for the first 10 years. Derrick's involvement in the military, his schooling, training for his subsequent career and later a job 100 miles from home typically kept us separated during the weeks and reunited on the weekends.

I kept busy working as a teacher during those years and we didn't discuss the issue of having children much. I do remember asking him about his feelings one day and he said 'not now' because he wouldn't be able to help me out much. I guess we thought we would have a child some day, yet we just kept postponing when we would try. In the meantime, our friends were having children. What really helped was that our best friends were unable to have children and they decided against adoption or medical treatment.

Also, my mind was usually preoccupied with serious medical problems that arose during that span of time. While I went on medication for Mitral Valve Prolapse, I also endured numerous surgeries for scar tissue buildup, a fibroid tumor and problems related to extreme bleeding that eventually led to a hysterectomy.

Meanwhile, fear became a great issue in my life. In fact, the panic attacks I experienced led me to investigate clinical help. Luckily it wasn't needed and the Lord used a great counselor and several Bible studies to lead me to a greater faith in Him and His provision. 'Divine Surrender,' a local study really helped me face difficult issues. I learned how to surrender my husband to the Lord, and I learned that the fear and anxieties I was experiencing were largely due to wanting control in all areas of my life.

Two other Bible studies helped me as well: 'Experiencing God' and a local infertility study by Christi helped me give up my dream of being a mom. The Lord got right to the point with me and I eventually accepted the concept that He loves me dearly and He is faithful.

As I look back on the events that have unfolded over the years, I see God's faithfulness in providing for us, especially when I look at how He moved us to a town in a different state where we are now happy as a family of two. We still have difficult times and the question 'How many children to you have?' continues to haunt us, however I have been able to answer quite simply that 'I was not able to have children, but being a teacher for a number of years makes me feel like I have had the blessing of many children.'

I know we will continually be answering this question especially now that Derrick and I are beginning our journey as business owners of a home tutoring service. I pray the Lord will continue to give us the ability to answer gracefully. I also pray that the Lord will forgive me when I do get upset and resent not having children or when I get upset with my husband for not wanting to adopt. At those times, opening the scripture is the best thing for me to do. Meditating on God's word... laying down at His feet and remembering His love for me is my reprieve.

I want to know Him better than I do now, because without Him I can do nothing. My point of view and my perspective on this issue would not have been what it is today if God had not intervened and opened the doors to life with Him. Otherwise, it would have been a life lived in fear. Second Timothy 1:7 continually reminds me, 'For God has not given us a spirit of timidity, but of power, love and discipline.'

> **"It is God who directs the lives of his creatures; everyone's life is in his power." Job 12:10 (TEV)**

Grieving is a Process

When it comes to the subject of infertility, I believe grieving is a given. First, we grieve the "attack" on our womanhood, hence the "i" word has reared its ugly head. Second, as we move on to fertility testing, both men and women grieve the idea of successful, natural conception. When a man finds out he is sterile, I would certainly guess he experiences grieving the loss of a precious part of himself and his family heritage.

The woman, on the other hand, grieves the "dream" of motherhood. She probably grew up picturing what her future family would "look" like; she probably expected a certain amount of children, she may have pictured in her mind what traits and characteristics they would have, and she may have even selected names for her dream children.

Obviously, once a couple loses a child the grieving process becomes an integral part of their lives. And last, an infertile couple that has surrendered their will for God's and chosen to continue life as a complete family grieves the "dream of parenthood."

The grieving process is natural, not shameful. I believe it is a process and I feel it is essential if you are going to be healthy human beings who are able to move on and accept the future God intends for you with open hearts, open minds, and your marriage in tact.

Glahn and Cutrer offer the following encouragement for couples facing infertility in their book. They understand the grieving process and explain it this way: *"Some people observe a childless woman and say to themselves, 'She needs to stop baby craving.' Would we expect a fire to stop itself? People to stop dying... rainfall to sit on the surface of the earth? In general, God instilled in women a need to bear and nurture children. So the tears an infertile woman cries simply validate the truth of what God said in Proverbs: Grieving over infertility and longing for that genetic link is normal.*

When righteous Hannah experienced infertility, she wept bitterly, felt 'greatly distressed,' described her self as oppressed, and wouldn't eat. Notice that God does not say to her, 'You shouldn't feel that way.'"

Glahn and Cutrer say that if infertility were an event, couples could grieve the loss and move on; but infertility is a process. Thus, grief may drag on for years. Many have described it as a roller coaster of hope and despair. *"Psychologists in one study asked infertility patients to rate the stress of infertility among stressful events ranging from 0-100, with the death of a spouse rating 100, divorce at 73, and the death of a close relative at 63. These patients rated the stress of infertility as sixth of 43 on the scale at 59.7. Another study indicates that fertility patients are second only to cancer patients in what they are willing to endure for a 'cure.'*

Some have identified a pattern to the stages of grief in mourning over lost dreams. One woman wrote, 'We discussed the grief process in my psychology class. Knowing each step helped me identify my feelings about infertility that seemed so intense each month. Categorizing them helped me to see that each was typical enough that someone had actually documented it as a normal part of coping,'" said the authors.

CHAPTER 10—OPENING YOUR EYES TO ABUNDANT BLESSINGS

The Stages of Grief

In Chapter 6 I mentioned that after witnessing many women's reactions to infertility, I noticed that each went through stages or processes. Glahn and Cutrer continue with their description of Stages of Grief:

1. Denial

The first 'stage' of grieving is denial. I [Bill Cutrer—a board-certified obstetrician/gynecologist and ordained minister] find it interesting and at times exasperating to watch how couples initially respond. Many begin with a form of denial attributing lack of 'success' to timing, stress, or other external factors. Rare indeed is the case in which timing alone is responsible, but most couples have a distorted understanding of the basics of physiology and human reproduction.

At the other end of the spectrum are those patients who, upon hearing a diagnosis of infertility, become depressed and hopeless before I order the first test. Patients describe their experience with denial as follows:

Mary. '*When my period started each month, I would tell myself, It's only spotting until the flow began. Then I reminded myself some women have a period the first month they're pregnant. Maybe I was pregnant, and I wouldn't know for another 28 days. I would memorize what each period was like to see if it was abnormal or different from the ones I'd had for the last 15 years. When I realized it was just like all the rest, I knew I wasn't pregnant after all.*

Unfortunately, this denial process took several days, starting a few days before my period when I would tell myself, I don't feel like my period is going to start. Maybe I won't have one! I guess the reason I never cried on the first day of my period is because I was denying that it was actually happening.'

Bobbie. '*I felt upset when a member of my church invited us to help lead a group for infertile couples. I told her in no uncertain terms, "I'm not infertile, I'm just having trouble getting pregnant!"*'

2. Anger

Cutrer points out that as couples continue to feel powerless, their frustration level builds. They often begin to express anger toward God, themselves, their spouses, other family members, friends, people with children, their doctors, and pregnant women.

Mary. 'Anger would follow a few days later and I would ask, "Why did God make this happen again?" I would get angry with myself as well, saying, If only we'd had sex every day instead of every other day... You can imagine what I said to myself after a friend told us, "The second ejaculate in one night has a higher concentration of sperm."

I began saying to myself, If only we hadn't been so tired—we should have done it twice a night this month. I got angry that I had consumed caffeine, NutraSweet®, taken cold tablets, and done all the things my pregnant friends' doctors put on their 'forbidden' lists. If only I hadn't done those things, I would have been pregnant.

Maybe I had been pregnant; then when I drank that hot chocolate, the caffeine killed the baby, and I miscarried—except it happened the same time my period was due, so I never knew it. I felt angry that millions of fourteen-year-old girls could get pregnant after one night at a party; I felt angry that fertile Myrtle from the office was pregnant; I felt angry, of course, about all the stupid, well-meaning comments I heard.'

Ann. 'I've read that anger turned inward is depression, and anger turned sideways is humor. That must be why I try so hard to see the humor in it all —I have a lot of anger. I told my husband I thought the reason it took so many millions of sperm to find the egg is because none would humiliate themselves by stopping to ask for directions.'

Barbara. 'After a church softball game, my husband and I went out with a friend who mentioned that someone we know was pregnant. He said he could understand that it was hard for me to hear the news, but I should be happy for her. I told him "I am." A few minutes later this was bugging me and I flat out said, "Don't ever challenge me on whether I'm happy for her. Of course I am. I'm just not happy for me." I felt compelled to make this clear.'

Part of the anger stems from frustration over a seeming loss of control. This loss of control dominates two realms. The first is the 'today' – the inability to manage daily schedules and emotions. The second is the future. Infertility makes it impossible to predict the future or to accomplish goals.

Julie. 'This morning I had planned to attend a seminar, but I can't go because I have to test my urine for the LH surge, which hasn't happened yet. This is so immobilizing. I wonder what working women do when they don't have private offices in which to set up a chemistry lab.'

Melanie. 'I take my chart to my doctor and get a progress report like a student would. Did I fill it out right? Did I have sex right? Did I ovulate well? Did my temperature do what it was supposed to do? Do I get a good grade this month?'

Often patients compensate for their 'loss of control' by educating themselves with medical information. Arming themselves with data makes it easier to manage their treatment, and it also helps them make informed decisions about when to stop.

Katherine. *'I was uncertain about my resources, and I craved information. I found every article on infertility I could in the Reader's Guide to Periodic Literature and in Christian periodicals. I studied every infertile woman in the Bible. For me, information made it easier to be in control of my treatment (control defined as having an influence over the outcome). I could ask more intelligent questions and not feel so helpless.'*

3. Bargaining

Cutrer says that from here, couples often move to 'bargaining,' or cutting deals with themselves and with God.

Mary. *'I tell myself I'll quit drinking caffeine forever— that will show that I really want a baby. I'll be preparing my body in the right way to nurture a child. I'll have sex more, or I'll have sex less, or I'll pray daily to show God that I mean business. I thought He would honor these bargaining tools. I thought He would look down and say, "Wow. She's willing to give up Pepsi. She loves Pepsi! I'll let her have a baby now that she'll give up what her taste buds crave." All that just made me feel worse when I didn't uphold my end of the bargain.'*

4. Desperation

Months of suppressed anger bring depression said Cutrer. This stems both from feeling helpless and the chronic strain of treatment.

Elizabeth. *'I cried. I was quiet. I lost my appetite. I withdrew from friends and group activities.'*

Maggie. *'My biological clock still has a lot of time left, by my mental clock is running down.'*

Jill. *'I hate going to the mall and walking past maternity shops. I used to loathe seeing pregnant women there until someone reminded me that any woman I see might have been through infertility. I could actually shop without falling apart after that. Of course, when I see a pregnant seventeen-year-old, it's hard to convince myself she tried for very long. Anyway, Pampers and pregnancy test commercials drive me to the mute button.'*

Some depression also stems from feelings of low self-esteem and decreased self-confidence. Fifty-five percent of women surveyed said they felt less self-confident after they learned of their infertility.

Beth. *'I had to go to work after my appointment. As I drove, big tears welled up in my eyes. I just wanted to head for home and cry. When I got to work, I called my husband and told him what the doctor said. I said, "You must feel like you got ripped off. When you married me, you thought we'd have a family and now you're not getting what you bargained for."'*

Robyn. *'You start to doubt your self-confidence during those many miles that stretch on and on. A woman who has been told she cannot bear children starts to wonder and doubt who she is as a woman. It's part of the process of working through a world that you never though you'd be a part of.'*

Guilt often accompanies feelings of low-esteem. This guilt may stem from prior sexual experiences, abortion, and contraceptive methods concludes Cutrer. Donna writes, *'Twenty years ago I had an abortion. Now I am going through the guilt and hurt of something I did years ago. Ironically enough, infertility has struck me with full force. My doctor tells me an infection, complications brought on by my 20-year secret, may be responsible for my fertility problem.'*

He says that others may feel guilty about delaying childbearing. Still others experience guilt for less tangible negative feelings in general: *'Many of my friends were pregnant,'* writes a patient who avoided baby showers. *'I didn't want to take away from their joy. With these mixed emotions I was unforgiving of myself for being selfish. I saw my response as less than Christ-like. I wanted all my reactions to be the way I perceived a perfect, godly woman to be. I wanted them to flow naturally and remain indefinitely. When they didn't, I thought, maybe that's why God's punishing me. I had to learn to forgive myself when I didn't react in the perfect Christ-like way, because He forgives me. He gives grace. He builds the bridge between who we are and who we want to be in Christ.'*

All this anger drives many couples to alienate themselves from painful situations, pregnant friends, and those who have made insensitive comments. Soon they feel that there's no one left who understands. They feel isolated. Their sources of outside support diminish, intensifying their need for intimacy at a time when each feels less capable of providing support added Cutrer.

Mary. *'I'm dreading the baby shower. I'm afraid conversation will turn to dilation, contractions, and Lamaze breathing. I can't relate; I can't participate; I can't even imagine what it feels like.'*

CHAPTER 10—OPENING YOUR EYES TO ABUNDANT BLESSINGS

Lara. *'I avoided church last Mother's Day, and I skipped two weeks ago because I found out about an infant baptism. In fact, last Sunday I checked the bulletin to make sure there wasn't a baptism next Sunday. There's a newlywed couple in our Sunday school class, and I'm so afraid she will show up in a maternity dress. I'll just lose it right then and there. I hate how this becomes something I focus on so much, but it's just so ongoing.'*

Cutrer noted that each month when her period comes, the wife usually feels a deep sense of loss. Yet she tells herself no loss has occurred. It's true that the couple has not actually lost a physical child, but the concept of a baby exists. They also realize they'll have to face at least one more month of tests, waiting, stress, expense, and uncertainty.

5. Mourning

Cutrer believes that when we cry, both our emotions and our bodies release tension, and privately sobbing for a lost dream actually provides a positive expression of sorrow.

Keith. *'It's a lot like when somebody dunks you too long—that deep ache, gripping your throat and then diving to your lungs. If you fight it, flailing and kicking, you might find air. But what if you don't? All that energy burned. The alternative feels a lot like suicide. The only way you can really conserve oxygen is to hold still, to surrender to the one holding you down, praying that he'll show some mercy and let you breathe. My wife and I want a baby real bad; sometimes I see her fighting for breath, flailing, and taking in water. So I jam my hands deep in my pockets, and I squeeze my eyes tight. I pray we don't drown.'*

Sally. *'I felt pain so severe that I was certain someone had torn an organ from my body, leaving in its place a gaping wound, a psychological hurt no one could ever see and few would even comprehend as little more than self-indulgence.'*

6. Acceptance

Eventually, couples that have worked through each stage of the process reach the point of acceptance, looking ahead more optimistically to alternatives teaches Cutrer. They begin to feel increased levels of energy and enthusiasm. Although the pain never disappears, it somehow becomes more manageable as they gain a renewed sense of purpose, even though they realize they may never bear a biological child. Often couples having the most difficulty getting to this stage are those with unexplained infertility and those who have conflict in their marriages or their families.

Debbie. *'I lost my five-year-old son to leukemia. Six months later we began trying again. That was four years ago. I have now put this into God's hands and taken a break, which has done me so much good – I haven't felt this good in years. I guess I went from the pain of losing a child to the pain of infertility, and now I feel like I have my life back.'*

Karen. *'I've had two failed in vitro cycles, so I understand the pain; but sometimes when going through infertility, it's easy to become so self-absorbed that we can't see anyone or anything else. If one in six couples of childbearing age is experiencing infertility, five of six are not. If I get bent out of shape at church on Mother's Day, why not dwell on the fact that those five in six women deserve to hear a Mother's Day sermon? Or why not spend the day feeling thankful for my own mother?'*

Cutrer concludes by reminding us that these comments present infertility in stages with specific sequencing. However, in general, grieving couples do not experience these reactions in the same order. Unique to infertility, the injection of hope at mid-cycle complicates the entire process.[1]

Did any of that sound familiar? It certainly did to me. Continue to go back and re-read these sections when you are feeling especially anxious, upset or depressed. Sometimes it helped me to read about other people's emotions and experiences so I didn't feel so alone, or like I was going crazy. I truly believe grief is part of the healing process.

If, on the other hand, you feel you are spiraling into a deep depression, make sure to go back and re-read God's love letters to you in Chapter 4. Also, read about how to fight off the enemy and how to resist the snare of footholds, strongholds and bondage in Chapter 5.

Dianne lost nine babies as she tried to provide a sibling for her son. Even though she was devastated along the way, the grieving commenced to a point that she could move on with her life in an optimistic manner: *"Tears still come. Sometimes you feel as though you are going in a vicious circle as each stage of grief comes along. You think you may have finished one cycle, and here it comes again.*

But the hopeless feeling fades away. Hope begins to come with each new day. You embrace God's promises, and you remember God loaned you a wonderful son. He even loaned you nine other babies for three or four months. They were created in your womb, and they were a vital part of you. Instead of being born full of vitality here on earth, they went straight to heaven to live with their heavenly Father who embraces them. All they have ever known has been peace and perfection. Our Father is their caregiver, and they have a secure place for eternity."

To the Child We Never Knew

We've tried to conceive of a child like you.
Your beautiful face, a mix of two.
With eyelashes that curl just like your dad,
And Mommy's red cheeks when you are mad.
Precious child, we love you so,
So much more than you'll ever know.
We pray each day for grace anew,
To grieve a child we never knew.

By Sarah Collier[2]

Blessing You is God's Gift!

Because the nature of infertility involves a lot of self-absorption and inner searching, grief is an inherent ingredient. It is easy to get so caught up in the whirlwind of tests, scheduled sex, buying groceries, paying the rent, more tests, more sex, bad news, feeding your pets... that you neglect the blessings surrounding you.

I want you to try something. When you wake up each morning, make it your goal to immediately fill your mind with these thoughts:

1. I have a committed partner, sent by God "to complete me," lying next to me. Many single women would give anything to be in my shoes.
2. I have my health—some people are experiencing dreadful disease and even eminent death.
3. I have a roof over my head, not everyone does.

4. God has provided warm clothing and food in my cupboards.
5. I have family and friends who love me and want to help me through this.
6. If you have a child, remind yourself that you've gotten to experience a miracle.
7. If you are going through testing, be thankful that you live in the age of technology.
8. If you are adopting, stop and pray for the birth parents and for the safety and welfare of your unborn child.
9. Last, remind yourself, *I have a bright new day, God's love and grace, forgiveness of my sins, and most importantly, salvation.*

I suggest that you start your day by reading Matthew 6:25-34 (NLT) which beautifully describes how God promises to provide for your needs: "*So my counsel is: Don't worry about things—food, drink, and clothes. For you already have life and a body—and they are far more important than what to eat and wear. Look at the birds! They don't worry about what to eat—they don't need to sow or reap or store up food—your Heavenly Father feeds them. And you are far more valuable to him than they are. Will all your worries add a single moment to your life?*

And why worry about your clothes? Look at the field lilies! They don't worry about theirs. Yet King Solomon in all his glory was not clothed as beautifully as they. And if God cares so wonderfully for flowers that are here today and gone tomorrow, won't he more surely care for you, O men of little faith?

So don't worry at all about having enough food and clothing. Why be like the heathen? For they take pride in all these things and are deeply concerned about them. But your Heavenly Father already knows perfectly well that you need them, and he will give them to you if you give him first place in your life and live, as he wants you to. So don't be anxious about tomorrow. God will take care of your tomorrow too. Live one day at a time."

Don't take these verses for granted. Think on what is positive, uplifting and beneficial first thing in the morning before your mind can start listing what you don't have. Throughout the day, rely on the Lord to keep your mind free of negative thoughts. And, look around—He created such beauty: the grandeur of the mountains, sunsets brimming with magnificent colors, white, frothy waves washed about seas of green, and of course, the rainbow—God's covenant with His loved ones. Thank him for your blessings; He deserves the credit.

Read how a lady named Karen took a step back to observe her world. She said, *"Because finances dictate so much of our lives in today's society, we are unable to proceed further with any options that have expenses associated with them. Therefore, we have come to realize that we will live a life without children. Every day I still question WHY God has chosen this path for my husband and me. It's a question I'm sure we'll never know the answer to.*

But the one big thing that has comforted me is the thought that we all must bear some kind of burden in our lifetime, and if this is the burden I must bear, then I will. I will because, even though I am not blessed with children, God has blessed me in so many other wonderful ways, and He will bless me in my life without children as well."[3]

I highly recommend that before you ask God for more blessings in your life, notice the daily blessings delivered directly from Him. The Israelites didn't and the consequences were heavy. *"They did not worship you despite the wonderful things you did for them and the great goodness you showered upon them. You gave them a large, fat land, but they refused to turn from their wickedness,"* (Nehemiah 9:35 NLT). Remind yourselves of what their punishment was!

Blessings Through Spiritual Gifts

If you are still suffering with any feelings of shame or disgrace, dispel them immediately. Disgrace is basically losing honor, respect, reputation, or feeling shame. Shame is rooted from guilt; remember, Chapter 2 instructed you that guilt, and therefore, shame and disgrace are not from God, they are planted in your mind by the devil.

Shame made me feel dirty about something I had no control over. If you need a practical way to rid yourself of this unhealthy feeling, try taking a bath or shower the next time you experience it. Make your self feel clean and watch the dirty water going down the drain forever. Let the dirt stay down with its creator and allow your self to feel spotless before your Creator.

Remember His grace. According to the Bible: *"grace is God's voluntary and loving favor given to those he saves. We can't earn it, nor do we deserve it."*[4] If God directs you to continue life as a complete family, hit your knees, turn your face up to the heavens and shout "thank you!" He has "opened and shut doors" to show you His will and because of your obedience, resounding peace and joy shall follow one way or another.

Furthermore, through His grace, God has blessed you with "spiritual gifts." They are special abilities given to each person by the Holy Spirit. They enable you to minister to the needs of the body of believers. A few include faith, hospitality, administration, wisdom, leadership, service, discernment, (see 1 Corinthians 12:8-11, Romans 12, Ephesians 4, 1 Peter 4:10, 11 to learn more).

Please take the time, right this minute, to go to Appendix B and complete the Spiritual Gifts Evaluation and determine what your top three gifts are. If you have taken this test before, go ahead and do it again – sometimes your gifts change. List them here:

1._____
2._____
3. _____

Now that you know what your special, God-given abilities are, learn more about how to apply them to your life. I am willing to bet they were placed in your life for a reason. For instance, my top three spiritual gifts (in order) are: 1) faith, 2) administration and 3) mercy. First, God gave me the trial of infertility; my *faith* was expanded immensely; through *administration*, I have been given writing skills; and *mercy* drives me to minister to all who experience this same trial.

Allow me to share examples of people in my life who have not "settled" for God's answer, but who have taken their spiritual gifts and embraced them for the sake of others:

Married friends of mine are missionaries. They tried to conceive for a short time and then realized that to be mobile for Christ, they had to be flexible. Children's schooling and medical needs often determine where a family lives, the focus is often on them, and in this case, being "tied down" so to speak was not their calling. However, God filled their needs by sending a Godchild into their lives whom they love, lead and encourage just like a son. In addition, in their own words, they have "spiritual children" all over the world that they adore.

Many, many of the ladies I have counseled over the years love children, so instead of giving birth to them or adopting them, God uses these beautiful ladies to teach them. Often the hugs, smiles, encouragement and attention they give children in their classrooms are the only hugs, smiles, encouragement and attention these children get in their lives. These ladies are given an opportunity to show Christ's love to a child. What could be more meaningful?

I have also witnessed many ladies who are incredible childcare facilitators, Sunday school teachers, youth group leaders, and even coaches. We have to remember that there are many children in this world today whose parents are unloving, uncaring, abusive, and even absent. God sends others who have a "heart" for children to their rescue.

Think about the children in your family. Do you have a particularly strong relationship with one of them? You may consider mentoring that child in morals, values, education, etc. Godchildren need mentoring as well. There may be a child on your block or in your community who needs someone to spend time with him or her so they can feel special. Look around, keep your eyes open and see where God leads you.

Dixie did and this is what she learned: *"I have come to terms with the fact that I will not contribute more members to my extended family. But that doesn't mean that I can't contribute to the enrichment of the new generation of nieces and nephews that I do have. I am an aunt, and although it is only a supporting role, why not make the best of it? Why not be the best aunt I can be?"*[5]

I have also met women who have experienced horrible disease and even mental problems in their lives, and they unselfishly chose to abstain from motherhood to save an innocent child from such anguish. Some "sickly" women I have met realize that their bodies are too fragile to go through childbirth and instead of risking the loss of their life and introducing an infant to a life without a mother, they too, decide to give up their dream of motherhood.

Some of these ladies utilize their "nurturing" instincts in these capacities: 1) Caring for animals at animal adoption agencies and rescue facilities. 2) Caring for plants in a green house. 3) Arranging flowers for a florist. 4) Visiting with or volunteering at a hospital, nursing home or "special needs" facility for children.

Ruth struggled with secondary infertility for 15 years. Instead of being mad at God, she gives Him credit for being faithful to her. *"I have journeyed on a road that I wouldn't wish on my worst enemy and yet I have not journeyed alone. Why did God choose this path for my life? Why has my son who would have made the most wonderful brother been left as an only child here on earth? I can't answer these questions. God knows why he chose this path for us.*

Over the years I have worked with the children's choir at church and I coached my son's swim team—activities that gave me an opportunity to have some impact on other children. If I couldn't have more of my own, I could still give love and attention to these children. We have also opened our home to four exchange students whom my son considers his brothers and sisters and I consider my daughters and sons. I may not have given birth to them, but I have helped to shape their lives."

Thank You

Even though we've waited for many years,
Thank you Lord, for being with us each step of the way.
Even though others are aborting babies,
Thank you Lord, for those who value human life.
Even though hurtful words are sometimes spoken,
Thank you Lord, for friends who seem to understand.

Even though we might not ever be a mom or dad,
Thank you Lord, for giving us good parents.
Even though we know no parental sacrifices,
Thank you Lord, for sending and sacrificing your Son.
Even though the pain is sometimes hard to bear,
Thank you Lord, for being the God of all comfort.
Even though we may never hear a child say, "I love you,"
Thank you Lord, for Your unconditional love.
Even though we may never fully understand why,
Thank you, Lord, for showing us this is part of Your Master Plan.

By Erica K. Skattebo[6]

Considering Your Spouse's Feelings

Unfortunately, many of us get caught up in "the chase" and neglect the foundation of our marriage—our spouse. I've mentioned that you should consider taking breaks during the journey to work on your marriage. Don't wait until you're on the other side of this "Grand Canyon" issue to look back and see how your partner is doing.

CHAPTER 10—OPENING YOUR EYES TO ABUNDANT BLESSINGS

Your spouse is a gift from God too. He is a blessing and a piece of the plan God designed for you long ago. Because men and women often react differently to the struggles infertility brings upon their marriage, it is important to take steps in understanding each other's feelings. Peoples and Ferguson describe reverse role-playing ideas that really opened my eyes to this concept. I hope it will help you understand your spouse's responses and emotions:

For the Husband:

- **If your wife finds out she did not get pregnant this month, see if you can understand how she feels by imagining that:**

When you were a young boy, you wanted to be on a team, you worked out for weeks, practiced with family and friends, ate the right foods, took vitamins, and so forth, and the day of the tryouts you did your best—in fact you thought you did great—but sadly you did not make the team.

- **When your wife cries all night long that her sister got pregnant, see if you can understand how she feels by imagining:**

When you were a teenager, all your friends had cars, and you badly wanted one also, but you just did not have enough money to buy it. So you asked your parents and grandparents for money, and even asked your sisters and brothers to contribute to your savings. One day when you came home from school, you saw a new, used car in your driveway. Convinced your parents had fulfilled your dream, you ran into the house cheering, screaming and jumping up and down that you finally could be like all the others. But you stopped dead in your tracks when you learned that your parents did not buy it for you, but gave it to your brother instead. They told you they felt you were just not ready yet.

- **When your wife gets so anxious waiting for the results of a pregnancy test that she cannot focus on anything else, see if you can understand how she feels by imagining:**

You felt pretty confident after you interviewed for your very first job. Everything went so well that you could hardly believe it. You wanted this job. It would offer you everything you dreamed of, everything you had worked so hard to prepare for. They told you they liked you and you had a good chance of getting it. But of course, they had to interview others and would let you know their final decision within a week or so. You sat by the phone every day hoping they would call and let you know so you could move on with your life.

- **When your wife is pregnant for six weeks and then has a miscarriage, see if you understand how she feels by imagining:**

You got the job of your dreams and everything was going along well: you finally had money in your pocket, so you bought yourself a car, rented an apartment, and even went on a vacation. One morning you walked into work happy and content, and your boss called you into his office. You figured it was about the promotion you expected to get; instead he told you the company was not happy with your performance. He fired you on the spot with no warning.

Now for the Wife:

- **When your husband tells you he is angry because you do not listen to his suggestions for how to solve your infertility problem, see if you can understand how he feels by imagining:**

When your best friend has a problem, she calls you every day to tell you how badly she feels, how her world has been destroyed. But each time you say something to help her see it from another perspective, she says you are wrong. You try to rephrase your suggestions so she can understand you, but she insists you still don't know what you are talking about.

- **When your husband says he is angry because no other problems besides the infertility seem important anymore, not even his problems see if you can understand how he feels by imagining:**

A friend of yours has a serious problem with a relationship. She had been dating her boyfriend for five years and they seemed really caring and loving of one another. She had told you many times that they would eventually be married, but then something happened and the relationship ended. And now she talks about it incessantly. No matter what the situation is, or the conversation is about, she always brings the subject back to her problem. She makes you feel as if your problems pale in comparison to hers. They are not even worth talking about. It is as if you don't exist.

- **When your husband tells you that getting pregnant is not the most important thing in the world, that you should move on and look at other ways to create a family, see if you can understand how he feels by imagining:**

Your sister calls for the fourth time today—the seventeenth time this week—to tell you about the same problem she has had forever. Her boyfriend is mean to her, never calls her when he is supposed to, never gets her presents or takes her out. But for some reason, she will not break up with him. You encourage her to move on, telling her that there are other fish in the sea. But she tells you she loves him and that she would do anything to get him to change. She knows it sounds stupid, but that is how she feels.

Peoples and Ferguson say that by switching roles, even momentarily you may be able to understand the frustration, loneliness, and disappointment your spouse is feeling.[7]

Blessed by Marriage

Your marriage is "put through the test" during infertility and I believe the best thing you can do is keep it strong. Your foundation has got to be secure. To obtain security, you must **pay attention to one another, maintain strong communication, and respect and trust each other.** As I have eluded, my husband and I didn't communicate about this issue and I ended up resenting him for not taking an active interest in our future family. I felt alone and I just wanted him to offer some encouragement, sensitivity and support for something that meant so much to me.

Here are some ways you can solidify the foundation of your lifelong investment: **Pay attention** to each other like you did when you were engaged and when you were newlyweds. Remind yourself of what attracted you to your spouse when you met. Think about the hobbies you used to enjoy together; revisit the short and long-term goals you made together.

If you have scrapbooks or photo albums collecting dust in the closet, get them out and reminisce about special memories you share together. Praying together is highly recommended to help you reconnect with each other and become more intimate in your bond. Plus, rekindle the home fires by the use of romance instead of a calendar.

Letter writing also helps. I articulate best this way, so when something is difficult for me to discuss with my husband, I write him a letter. Sometimes he writes back and addresses my issues and other times my letter induces **communication** between us. Leaving little, love notes in his lunch, car, drawers, etc. is also a fun way to remind him that he's love. Perhaps you'll want to try it sometime.

Respect comes in many forms. When it comes to infertility, if the problem lies with the wife, there's a good chance the husband will feel relieved. If the problem lies with him, this can be extremely insulting to his masculinity. Be prepared to be supportive in ways most appropriate for him.

Respect also comes from listening and avoiding blaming, name calling or inappropriate questioning. Colossians 3:8 warns us to *"But now you must rid yourselves of all such things as these: anger, rage, malice, slander, and filthy language from your lips."* One mistake I have often made and I heed you to avoid is pouting and holding a grudge. I knew about this verse in Ephesians: *"In your anger do not sin: Do not let the sun go down while you are still angry, and do not give the devil a foothold"* (4:26, 27) and I didn't obey. I wanted the last word, so I would be angry for days and give my husband the silent treatment. Did it work? Never!

Trust is the cornerstone of your union. Stop and think of how confident you felt on your wedding day. Make a list of the ingredients that went into that assurance and keep repeating it day after day, year after year.

Let's go a step further and see what God Almighty says about marriage in His Word:[8]

Genesis 2:18-24	Marriage is God's idea
Genesis 24:58-60	Commitment is essential to a successful marriage
Genesis 29:10, 11	Romance is important
Matthew 19:6	Marriage is permanent
Ephesians 5:21-23	Marriage is based on the principled practice of love, not on feelings
Ephesians 5:23, 32	Marriage is a living symbol of Christ and the church
Hebrews 13:4	Marriage is good and honorable

Because there are so many references to marriage in the Bible, I am lead to believe that God knew it would be difficult and in His loving way, He chose to aid us with great advice. Consequently, Satan, our adversary, chooses difficult areas of our lives to attack. Marriage and fertility seem to be obvious targets. Protecting your marriage and your "help mate" are important to God and should be just as important to you.

How to Strengthen a Damaged Marriage

It is ironic to me that two people unite in marriage normally with the intention of eventually "growing" their family unit by the addition of offspring only to realize later that the inability to create said offspring is what strained their union.

CHAPTER 10—OPENING YOUR EYES TO ABUNDANT BLESSINGS

Is that you? Roxanne Griswold shares great tips on solidifying a troubled marriage in her article titled, "Preserving Your Marriage When Infertility Pulls it Apart." She asks: *"Is there strife in your marriage? Disagreement? Has infertility divided your hearts, your decisions, and even your love for each other? Maybe you're confident a specific medical technique could increase your likelihood of conception, but your husband is uncomfortable with the idea. Or maybe you long to build your family through adoption, but your wife is persistent about having a biological child. Whatever has alienated and divided your hearts as a result of your childless condition, I believe there are three essentials for adding harmony and enrichment back to your marriage:*

1. Make Your Partner Your Priority

Griswold said her conversations with her husband were consistently tainted with dissatisfaction over infertility. Every day it was the same thing. Days turned into months and months turned into years. *"Not only had I struggled with infertility for sixteen years,"* she said, *"but I had lost six babies to ectopic pregnancy, and experienced two failed adoptions as well. I felt I had every reason to bemoan my circumstances, but the more I talked about it, the more frustrated my husband, Bob, became. My unhealthy fixation with having a baby translated to my husband that he wasn't as important."*

Griswold found the best solution to her unhappiness and her husband's frustration was deliberately putting his needs before hers... *"like the times I laid aside my agenda to organize the garage, wash his truck, or show interest in his woodworking hobby. It wasn't long before the tension subsided and my husband reciprocated with his love and appreciation,"* she shared.

"Putting Bob's needs first has reaped a huge return on my investment," Griswold said. *"Instead of depleting my marriage, it has built lasting intimacy. Instead of feeling robbed of my 'right' to motherhood, it has caused me to see my spouse as a gift from God. He is my family (as well as my two stepsons). Having children would be merely an extension of that family. Just as children are a part of me, my husband is a part of me. 'This is now bone of my bones and flesh of my flesh,' (Genesis 2:23)."*

Griswold says that when we feel deprived of a family, we have forgotten the gift God has already given in our spouse. She reminds you not to let infertility rob you of this realization. Moreover, don't let it forfeit a deeper relationship with your spouse or your Creator. Instead, acknowledge your gratitude to God for this special gift by laying aside your agenda for them. In time, you will reap a precious return on your investment.

2. Reserve Time for mutual prayer

Griswold says that if you carve out a specific time in the day when the two of you can meet God together, you will experience some of the richest, most intimate times of fellowship and communication. In fact, you will actually look forward to it.

"Unfortunately, it took severe hardship before Bob and I realized the need for mutual prayer. But an amazing change took place in our marriage when we made that daily commitment every morning. We were less tense with each other and about our circumstances, and more in sync with God's will for our lives. Prayer continues to knit our hearts closer in spiritual intimacy," she shared.

Griswold teaches that prayer is not only a time to commune with God, but to be open with each other. Prayer is a forum that allows you the opportunity to be real and honest before the Lord and your spouse. Prayer will also give you the privilege of witnessing God's dramatic answers. *"I have seen it in my own life. God honors the couple that is steadfast in prayer. As you see God's faithfulness in the little things, you will be moved to trust more deeply for the bigger, more impossible things. You will conclude that if God cares about the insignificant details of your life, surely He will take the utmost care concerning the deeper issues – like your infertility. Together as a couple you will discover a simple, childlike faith that leads to a deeper level of trust in the Lord, and each other,"* she said.

3. Plan Surprises

"Bob always seemed to have a spontaneous streak that had a way of quickly raising my spirits. I remember the time he carefully planned my surprise trip to the Grand Canyon! Every discouraging thought about my infertility quickly dismissed itself that week at the Grand Canyon. Bob's thoughtful, caring ways carried me through, and sparked a new sense of appreciation for the gift God gave me in my spouse.

I've reasoned that if small children were there that season of my life, quite possibly I would never have experienced such fun-filled adventures and sublime spontaneity in my marriage. Moreover, because we've been free to enjoy each other through the years, there is richness to our relationship, and a zest that comes from spending quality time together, Griswold said.

She adds that it's important that you don't allow a busy schedule to cloud these special times with your spouse. *"And you don't have to spend a bundle to have fun together. Sometimes at the spur of the moment, Bob and I will leave work, and take a pleasant drive through the Smoky Mountains to our cabin, or through the Cherohala Skyway. Other times, we might play a game of Scrabble®, or watch a good movie together. The key is spending time together, and going out of your way to make that time special."*

Griswold adds practical ways you can add spontaneity to your marriage, even when infertility is dragging you down:

1. Send a love letter, card, or e-mail at work expressing your love, gratitude, appreciation, and praise.

2. Make it a point to compliment your spouse at least once every day, especially in front of others. Maybe you could mention how well he handled a difficult situation, or applaud him on a new accomplishment. Maybe you could tell her how beautiful she looks in that new dress – or better yet – buy her one! Either way, a compliment goes a long way.

3. Plan a little weekend trip for just the two of you – something that would be special and within your financial reach.

4. Rekindle the romance in your marriage by preparing your husband's favorite meal complete with candlelight, wine, and soft music. Husbands, you could do the same for your wife and really surprise her!

5. If you are undergoing treatment, take a break from it – set aside a designated time to just enjoy your marriage. Choose intimacy for romance, not for the sole purpose of pregnancy.

6. Bring back your fondest memories by looking together at photo albums of your childhood, of while you were still dating, or from your first year of marriage. Designate a date when you could relive happier times by revisiting the places you did before. For Bob and me, it was Maui, Hawaii, where we spent our honeymoon. Going back refreshed and revived us from the doldrums of hardship, while creating new memories.

7. Get involved in a joint outreach. Bob and I work together with our church youth group – comprised of more than 250 kids. This has truly added spice to our relationship. Not only does it make us feel young again, but also together we are making a lasting difference in the lives of these kids. Ministry gives you an incredible sense of meaning and purpose. Without a doubt, it has unified, strengthened, and blessed our marriage beyond measure.

Griswold concludes by adding: *"Don't let your childless condition rob you of the abundant life Jesus promised (John 10:10). And don't let it squelch a healthy, happy, vibrant marriage. If you will set in motion these practical, yet biblical principles, you will be simply amazed by the harmony and enrichment it adds to your relationship, even when children are a distant dream. Don't wait until that dream is fulfilled; start now by loving the family God has already given you in your spouse."*[9]

That's right—when you married you became a family, period. Sheri and her husband spent five years enduring tests, surgeries, ultrasounds and Artificial Inseminations. She says that she would cry and cry each month her period came. *"My husband could never understand. He was always disappointed too, but never like I was. He tried to be understanding and be sensitive, but he just wanted me to pick myself up and keep going, and I just wanted to crawl in to bed and die.*

For me, it was shameful. I was a woman who couldn't do what women are supposed to— make beautiful babies. I couldn't give that to my husband. There were many times I contemplated leaving him for HIS sake so he would still have plenty of time to find a real woman who could give him the family he longed for. Thankfully, God gave me a man who wouldn't stand for me walking out the door over something like that.

Sometimes infertility feels like it's ripping your marriage apart— sometimes it makes you feel like you have a connection other couples couldn't possibly comprehend."

Moving on as a Complete Family

Choosing to move on as a complete family is a very big decision for a couple. (Notice I didn't use the word "childless" or "child-free." I prefer the word "complete" because our mate makes us whole.) I admire this decision because it involves surrendering to God's will. This last "stage" of grief is no "booby prize," it is the green light to move on.

You may move on as a family of two or three, yet the end result must be acceptance. Ruth shares: *"My secondary infertility is always with me, although I am reconciled to my situation. My infertility formed me into who I am today. It formed my son into who he is and also my husband. My life is very different than I had planned! God chose this path for us—and I am now okay with it!"*

Moving on and creating new goals and aspirations is key, as well as giving God the continued direction with your life that *He already has*! As you could see from her testimony, Karen and her husband, Derrick, are doing just that. It will take time and it won't happen overnight. You must be realistic and give yourself a break. You've provably been dedicated to this single goal for years I would guess, and it will take time to refocus. Also, shed the "infertile identity" that has probably haunted you and graduate to a new realm of your life.

Tammy did, and she learned a lot about herself: *"So many times we think that the only 'happy ending' to an infertile couple's struggle comes when God blesses them with a child. But what about the couple for which God has different plans... a plan in which the couple remains a family of two? Is this couple any 'less blessed' or unfulfilled? Being a complete family after years of infertility can be a fulfilling life that honors God, and a life that He desires for some couples.*

Several months have passed since my husband and I reached the three-year mark in our struggle with infertility. We now feel that God is leading us to be a family of two, which is not second or third best, but may be THE best that God has in mind for us. There are times when I struggle, thinking that the world around us does not see us as a 'real' family. I am learning, though, to be less concerned about what the world thinks. (Believe me, this is a stretch for me!) I am focusing more and more on whom I am in Christ and how He sees me. He loves and values me whether I am a mom or not."[10]

The Van Regenmorter's feel there is nothing immoral in choosing to live positively while childless! If you are not able to have children biologically and you do not sense the Lord leading you toward adoption, please remember: There is nothing wrong with an infertile couple remaining a family of two.

"Be prepared, however!" they say. *"There will be those who will say, 'you can't give up trying to get pregnant. I'm sure there must be something more your doctor can do!' Do not permit anyone to make you feel guilty because you do not have children. Resist the influence of others who urge you to continue medical treatment long after you and your spouse have reached your financial or psychological limits. Do not be pressured by others to achieve a pregnancy by an assisted reproductive technology that is objectionable to you.*

Others may say to you, 'I can't imagine living in a big home like you have and not filling it with children. Why don't you just adopt?' As adoptive parents ourselves, we believe that adoption is a wonderful choice. We believe it was God's plan for us to begin our family through adoption. But adoption is not for everyone. It is a calling from God."

The Van Regenmorters are correct in advising people not to adopt a child just because others think that's what you should do. You should never adopt a child out of guilt because you think it is somehow your burden in life to provide a home for children, whether you want to or not. Adopting for such reasons is neither fair to the child, nor to yourselves!

"Contrary to popular opinion, God has never indicated that children are a necessary prerequisite for happiness or fulfillment in marriage. In the opening pages of Genesis, God declares, 'A man will leave his father and mother and be united to his wife and they will become one flesh.' There is a period at the end of that sentence! A Christian husband and wife can find fulfillment in each other and in service to the Lord, with or without children," they urge.

"A couple without children can develop many avenues for Christian service, which may not be easy for couples with children to pursue. They could 'adopt' some disadvantaged or special needs children in their community, such as in the 'big brother' or 'big sister' programs. Infertile couples could become 'children' to older persons who have no children to care for them. We know a childless couple that opens their home to children who come into their community to attend the local school for the deaf. Another couple is involved with a local ministry called 'Moses' in which adults take groups of young people on service project trips.

We are not suggesting that a childless couple deny the hurt that being childless may bring. It is never safe or wise to deny real pain and disappointment, but a childless couple must not let the pain dominate. The Christian couple must not allow infertility to rob them of the joy God intended them to have in a relationship with Him and the partner whom He has given,"[11] concluded the Van Regenmorters.

The goal is to find satisfaction with your life so the desire for what you don't have will not rob you of the opportunity to enjoy what you do have. This woman sums it up best: *"I remember the day our lives changed forever because of one trip to the doctor's office. My husband and I had been married eight years and had decided we were ready to begin our family. I was not prepared for the news that would bring a contrary plan. After unsuccessful conception, we were told that I had PolyCystic Ovary Syndrome (PCOS).*

CHAPTER 10—OPENING YOUR EYES TO ABUNDANT BLESSINGS

My husband and I prayed and waited for months, which turned into years, for direction. The answer always seemed to be the same for both of us—acceptance. We would not pursue infertility treatments of any sort, nor would adoption be a possibility. We instead chose a focus that was completely on God—being a family of two. I found as months rolled by that God was changing my heart's desires. I found more and more that I wanted HIM above all else. He had replaced the desire for a baby with a desire for an intimate relationship with Him.

I know that in the years ahead, there will be special challenges. But I know that God is already there. Childless couples have no less a potential for joy and happiness than couples with children. It is all in our responses to the circumstances in which we find ourselves. We can either allow God to pick up the pieces and form a more brilliant picture than we thought possible, or we can stagnate for years, trying to make the same broken pieces fit into a picture that is not meant for us."

In my opinion, you just read an awesome example of a woman desperate for God. I truly admire her!

Rise Up My Child

Rise up and walk my child!
Rise up and walk anew.
Rise up and dance my child!
Your freedom is calling you.
Rise up and sing my child!
Utilize the voice I've given you.
Rise up and speak my child!
Remember: "I've anointed you!"
Arise my child!
Live life again!
I am the life that possesses you!
Think no more that you've got no home.
It's just an illusion that you're all alone.
Look around without a frown.
Invite a smile from a simple passerby.
I died and rose so that you would be free!
So stop the flow of hopelessness.
It's not reality.
Creativity is a gift that I've given you.
Reach out to humanity utilizing the gift.
Flow through your life confident and bold!
Use the gift of creativity to revive thirsty souls.

Copyright, October 1999, Portia A. Kennard, RN
(Used with permission.)

"You have given me your salvation as my shield. Your right hand, O Lord, supports me; your gentleness has made me great. You have made wide steps beneath my feet so that I need never slip."
Psalm 18:35-36 (NLT)

Chapter Eleven–Feeling Desperate for God

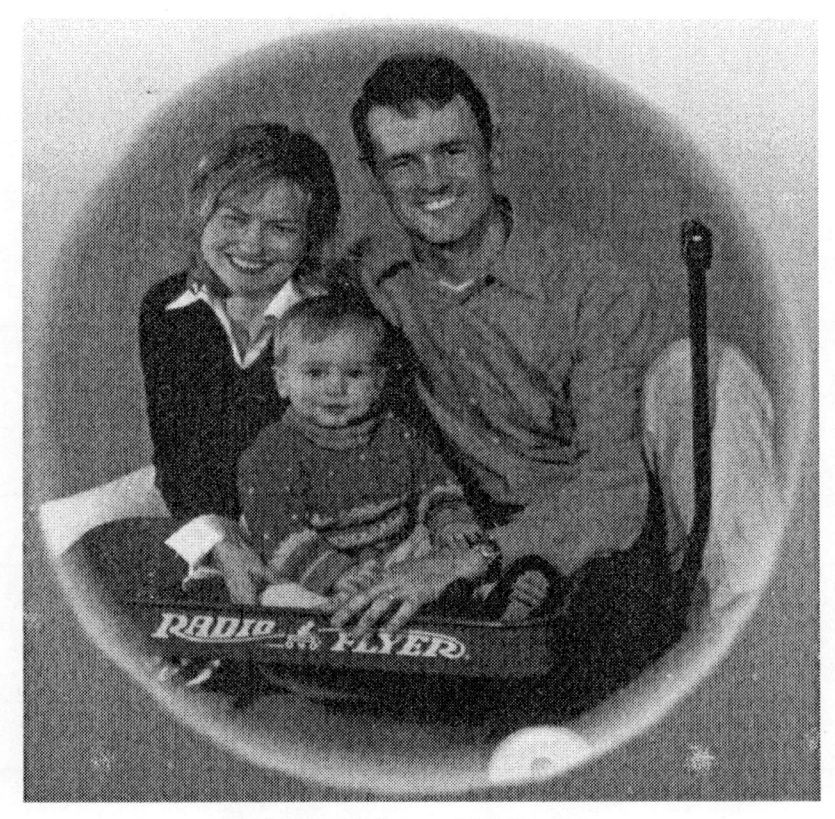

Christine, John and Little John

-Keeping Up Your Shield
-Examining Your Purpose for Living
-Blessings in Disguise

Chapter Eleven–Feeling Desperate for God

1. Do you feel desperate for God now? Yes or No? If no, what will it take until you humble your self and surrender your will for His?
___
___
___

2. List any new goals you have set for yourself recently:
___
___
___

3. List any new goals you and your hubby have set together or any hobbies you are considering together:
___
___
___

4. Where do you see yourself five years from now? (i.e. What plans do you have? What things do you want to change, etc.?)
___
___
___

5. How have you grown from this experience?

6. How has your relationship with Christ changed?

7. Do you look at trials differently now? Yes or No? If so, have your views changed?

8. Do you have any intentions or plans to help other couples going through this struggle? Yes or No? If so, please describe how:

9. What stage of grief are you currently in?

CHAPTER 11—FEELING DESPERATE FOR GOD

10. What is your purpose for living? Has it changed since you've experienced this trial? Please explain:
_____
_____
_____

11. What is your favorite verse?
_____
_____
_____

12. Please write it out for future reference:
_____
_____
_____

Recommended Reading:

Psalm 37:23-24   Mark 12:28-31
Romans 8:35-39   Ephesians 3:17-19
Colossians 1:16b   James 1:17

Look up these final verses and fill in the blanks:

Psalm 18:35: *"You gave me your _____ of victory, and your right _____ sustains me; you stoop down to make me great."*

Matthew 6:33 (NLT): *"So don't be anxious about tomorrow. God will take care of your tomorrow too. Live one _____ at a time."*

"Why *Did God Create me?"*
Answer #10 —A barren womb forces you to examine your purpose for living.

Chapter 11–Christine's Story

The despair of infertility is a slow, aching process. Baptisms, friends getting pregnant, baby showers, and Mother's Day became unbearable for me. Every year got worse and worse. Eventually I had to remove myself from those situations because they were just too painful for me. I had no other coping mechanism— just avoidance.

At first, my religion was not a means of support I chose. Each time I went to church I left feeling empty and worthless. Seeing so many families left me feeling like I was being punished because I could not have my own. I did use the church's resources to see a fertility specialist who was located far away from my home. I ended up having endometriosis surgery, as well as daily ultrasounds for one entire cycle. My husband and mother both stayed with me, but there was a short time when I was by myself.

During that period I went to church every morning before my ultrasound to pray. One Saturday, I went to confession before church and expressed to the priest that I was bitter and angry at God because He hadn't given me a child. The priest told me that God gives everyone special gifts and He doesn't give everyone the same gifts. He told me to be content with the gifts that God had given me. I was mortified. All I heard was that God might not choose to give us the gift we longed for. This haunted me for many years; all my thought processes revolved around what this man had said because he was my closest messenger from God.

While I was on Clomid for six months I did become pregnant for the very first time. My husband and I were in disbelief. Unfortunately our elation lasted less than one day because I developed very painful abdominal cramping and knew something was very wrong. We later learned I had experienced ectopic pregnancy. This is when the fetus tries to develop in the tubes instead of the uterus. Internal bleeding starts when the fetus outgrows the small tube. Because this can be life threatening, I had abdominal surgery immediately because of internal bleeding.

Physically it was a difficult, slow recovery. I remember feeling like I wanted to die, and I had no hope. I just could not understand why God would let me become pregnant and then take that precious life away. I again felt like a failure and I questioned whether I was being punished.

CHAPTER 11—FEELING DESPERATE FOR GOD

After dealing with infertility for four years and the ectopic pregnancy, I sank to rock bottom. I felt that we had done everything we could to make the best decisions and do all the right steps in trying to have a baby. I was finally to a point that I could do no more. I had to take steps to heal the pain. Very few people could help me and those who helped the most were those who had been through the same experiences.

Sometimes they were strangers to us, however, their advice always lead me in the right direction. My friends were supportive, but in large groups, I felt overwhelmed. I felt like everyone was feeling sorry for me. My family was positive, but I always felt like they thought I was trying too hard, or going to extreme measures to have a baby.

In order to go on with my life, I had to re-focus on myself. The purpose was to get my life back. I had to get off the roller coaster of rising expectations and dashed hopes. I had to deal with my feeling of anger and depression. I had to stop the relentless focus on my menstrual cycles, hormone levels, and numerous tests.

I had to learn to live in the present, with my mind and heart, and senses fully engaged. I never gave up hope I just had to put it aside. I realized that relationships with friends, family, work and marriage all suffer because of infertility. The best thing I ever did to help myself deal with this trial was learning to concentrate on helping myself.

I was no longer angry and bitter at God. I just had to have faith. Before I got to that point it never seemed like faith was enough, or perhaps it didn't work according to my timetable. I had to believe God would let it all be okay. My fears of being punished were gone and I finally understood what the priest had said to me. I finally took his advice and decided to focus on the gifts God had given me and I learned to be content with those gifts.

It finally clicked in my mind that God had given me a wonderful family, devoted friends, a wonderful husband, a beautiful marriage and a good career. I had to find the strength to focus on those gifts and release control of my life.

This freedom allowed me to pray again, but this time I was listening. Somehow I opened myself up and felt an inner peace that helped me go on with my life. This required surrender on my part. I actually felt God guiding me to press on, and my feelings of loneliness disappeared.

I reached out to a wonderful priest who was our pastor when my husband and I were in college. I wrote him a letter questioning him about God's plan. He said that God's plan for our lives is that we use the gifts and talents that we have, live in openness to divine love, and know that He is with us in the midst of all the difficulties we may experience. He added that these problems range from family problems, illness, financial issues, and even to more sensitive issues such as infertility.

He also said that perhaps God was calling us to share our married love, our generative love, in other ways. Once we heard this advice, we realized that God might have been opening our hearts to becoming parents in alternative ways such as adoption or IVF.

We opted for IVF and our first son was born two years ago to the day after I had my ectopic pregnancy loss. Two years later I became pregnant without the use of alternative methods. God did plan to "grow" our family. I believe He used those terrible years to teach my husband and I to cherish each other, to wait on God's timing, and to listen when we pray.

"...let us run with perseverance the race marked out for us."
Hebrews 12:1b

Keeping Up Your Shield

When I was writing this book, I was frustrated on a weekly basis by problems. They came in the form of physical ailments, financial problems, emotional issues, equipment problems, etc. I wanted to throw in the towel and admit defeat. I told myself this book just wasn't meant to be.

Then it hit me – this book *was* pre-ordained. It contained information intended to lead souls to Christ; it held within it suggestions and tips that would help hurting women; it emphasized a strong foundation in Christian marriages; it taught about surrender to the Lord; it was exactly what Satan hates. He wanted to force me to give up by inundating me with his fiery "missiles." I knew one thing: the enemy was threatened and therefore, the proverbial show had to go on!

The reason I'm telling you this, is because I want you to be aware of his schemes. Once you and your husband reach the point when you feel you are heading in the path God has chosen for you, peace and joy will return to your lives... for a while. Then what happens? Calamities in the forms previously mentioned! Once you are aware of the enemy's mischief, you can prepare yourself.

These calamities remind me of a sermon Pastor Mercer gave in June of 2003, titled, "What Will Satan Do About Your Success?" He said that the enemy reacts to our good fortune or peaceful periods with "strategies." I agree. It's no coincidence that on the way home from church something said will cause a family to argue. It's not just bad luck when you wake up sick the day you and your non-Christian friend are scheduled to have lunch together either.

That's also what happened to Barnabas and Saul (Paul), in the book of Acts 13-14. They were sent on the first missionary journey along with John Mark, who served as their assistant. In his sermon, Pastor Mercer taught that on this trip, the disciples experienced success eight ways and Satan reacted by attacking in eight ways: logistically, by false religion, by jealousy and slander, by persecution and oppression, by idolatry, attempted assassination, by confusion, and by exhaustion. The disciples were courageous and committed, therefore they responded to the enemy's schemes with persistence and moved on to spread the gospel to many.

You can read about that trip on your own, but for now I want to translate that insightful sermon into terms you can relate to. I've taken the eight attacks of Satan listed above and inserted them into scenarios related to infertility. I then inserted the eight correct responses Pastor Mercer said the Apostles used when they were hit with calamities. I want you to be as successful as they were when you are attacked. Here's how:

1. Logistical Attack—Let's say you and your husband pray about seeing a specialist 90 miles away. You feel led to go, so you book an appointment. On the way, your car breaks down. Your first reaction is *maybe we misunderstood and God was trying to tell us this wasn't his plan?* Pastor Mercer would tell you the correct response is: "**Deal with the problems and overcome.**"

2. Attacked by False Teachings—After two miscarriages, you find out you are pregnant with triplets. You're both ecstatic! Then the doctor cautions you that there may be a problem with two of the babies who share the same sac. He gives you three choices: 1) Keep all three babies and risk miscarriage or a difficult pregnancy, 2) have a pregnancy reduction, or 3) abort the pregnancy. You are both frightened by the news.

To make things worse, the doctor calls you into his office and pressures you to opt for the pregnancy reduction. You try to explain that you don't believe in abortion even if killing one or two of the babies would save one baby's life. I pray that none of you experience this horrendous scenario, however if you do, remember you are being attacked. According to Pastor Mercer, the correct response to this attack is: "**Be alert and confront it (the false teachings).**" In other words, do your homework ahead of time and consider moral issues in advance so you can make good decisions when the time comes. (By the way, this has happened to a couple I read about and all three babies were born healthy!)

3. Attacked by Jealousy and slander: Let's say you've been married for eight years and you've spent four of those years going through the infertility journey. Finally, you decide as a couple to relinquish your testing schedules and move on as a complete family. The mood in your home changes – it's like a burden is lifted and you both experience peace, happiness and tranquility for the first time in a long time. Spontaneity returns to your lives and your marriage prospers.

You decide to make a brief announcement to your families at Christmas and the news is not taken well. It's as if your loved ones preferred the two of you down in the pits with them and they are jealous of your renewed happiness. Soon you hear false rumors your sister-in-law is spreading. Even though this scenario sounds absurd, it happens. So, be prepared. Pastor Mercer says that in this form of attack the correct response is to: "**avoid bitterness and resentment – ignore the situation and move on**."

4. Attacks by Physical Persecution and Oppression: Let's say you and your hubby are driving to your infertility care group; you are going to announce your pregnancy and you both are bursting with joy. The drive seems long as you anticipate the gang's faces after they hear the great news.

Upon arrival your husband stands and makes the big announcement: you two are the first ones to have your prayers answered!! Dead silence. No one moves to hug you. Their mouths are dropped open and they show no signs of happiness for you. Now they are distressed and so are you. Pastor Mercer reminds us that the apostles chose to "**respond creatively**" when they were attacked. It's important to remain humble in the presence of oppression. Whatever you do, make sure to avoid pity parties. You may have to "graduate" from a care group and/or make new friends.

5. Satan Attacks By Using Reverse Psychology So Others Idolize You: Let's use a different scenario centering on an infertility care group. You are the oldest members of your care group and hence, you've experienced infertility the longest. Because the other members are younger they can't afford IVF. You and your groom decide to go for it and the gang is right there beside you. They excitedly help you with every detail as if they were going through the procedure themselves.

Afterward, they all gather to hear the results—you're pregnant! You are suddenly the heroes. Everyone in the room is congratulating you, admiring

CHAPTER 11—FEELING DESPERATE FOR GOD

your courage and wishing they were in your shoes. You both are so excited that you bask in the adoration. Pastor Mercer cautions you to be wise to Satan's trickery. He says the correct response is to **"clarify."** In humility, deflect the glory to God.

6. Attacks by Attempted Assassination: You and your mate have thrown in the towel and decided to move on as a complete family. You're both very comfortable with the decision, until one day when your doctor calls out of the blue indicating that one more test might provide the answer to your prolonged infertility. Your husband is fed up. All you want him to do is go in for one more semen analysis and he refuses.

You ask him, *"Am I really asking too much?"*

"Yes!" he snaps.

"I keep telling you I've had enough. All you talk about is tests. It's like your concentration on having a baby has overshadowed everything in your life—including me and my needs," he screams.

Pastor Mercer says that during periods of success, be careful to watch your marriage and your relationships. He says the correct response to this attack is **"gratitude."** Perhaps it's time to take a break and concentrate on the gift of marriage.

7. Satan Attacks by Developing Confusion: Picture yourself in a women's Bible study at church and no one else in the group is infertile. You are frustrated when you can't relate with them as they share about their families or problems with their children. You begin to feel confused as to why God placed you in this group, however, you feel compelled to stay. The leader is an excellent teacher and you learn a lot. Your faith grows and friendships blossom.

After three years, the leader announces that her husband has been offered a promotion in another state and they will be moving soon. She explains that you are all in a place to lead groups of your own now. A week later, a church representative calls you and asks you to lead a Bible study on Tuesday mornings. Notice when Satan is trying to develop confusion in your life. Instead of letting him keep you down, Pastor Mercer would say, **"develop leaders."**

8. Attacked by Exhaustion: You and your husband have spent 10 years struggling with infertility. Your marriage has been tested; your faith has been tested; your body has been poked, cut on and jabbed; and still your arms are empty. One day he comes to you and says, *"Honey, I need to take a break. I'm not telling you that I don't want a baby and I'm not telling you that I won't be supportive if you want to resume testing later, but for now, I believe it's in our* *best interests to take a break from baby making."* According to Pastor Mercer, the apostles got to a point when they needed to **"rest"** and when you reach a point of exhaustion, the correct response would be the same.

These are just a few examples. Learn from Paul and his travelling companions about overcoming obstacles by reading about them in the Book of Acts. There are many ways the enemy will try to frustrate you, railroad you or beat you down. Satan is crafty, he thinks he's pretty smart. But, he cannot read your mind. He can't be in all places at all times. He is not all powerful, but God is! It's a good thing you have Him on your side!

Keep up your faith. Keep praying and keep reading your Bible. The evil one loves to shoot arrows at your heart, so keep your "breastplate of righteousness" in place. Also, keep your "shield of faith" up to divert his deadly missiles!

Examining Your Purpose for Living

I believe that at some point everyone wonders why God put them on this green earth. I believe the answer lies in the Great Commission where Jesus told the 11 to *"go and make disciples of all nations"* in Matthew 28:18-20. Each of us is now an ambassador of Christ and our purpose is to tell others of His love for them.

This trial you are undergoing very well may be the "testimony" you share with an unsaved person some day. God's intention is to use your weaknesses for His glory, right? Perhaps you will share techniques you've learned such as reading the Word, praying, and surrendering with someone and make a great impact on their spirituality.

In the meantime, you may be at a point of frustration because you've been prevented from fulfilling your purpose as a mother. You've probably cried out *Why am I here God?* just like Christine did. I truly doubt God's answer would be: I made you to become a pharmacist, or a doctor, or a florist, or a nurse. I don't believe He put you here necessarily to become a wife or mother for that matter. Although, these areas of your life could possibly lead to your purpose.

You will find answers to this question in the book *The Purpose Driven Life*, by Rick Warren. I highly recommend that you read it. Warren explains that God is not just the starting point of your life; he is the **source** of it. To discover your purpose in life you must turn to God's Word, not the world's wisdom. He says that according to the Bible, *"It's in Christ that we find out* *who we are and what we are living for. Long before we first heard of Christ and got our hopes up, he had his eye on us, had designs on us for glorious living, part of the overall purpose he is working out in everything and everyone,"* (Ephesians 1:11Msg).[1]

Nikki and her husband, Jason, read the book and realized life is not all about them, it's about letting God work His purpose *through* them.

Nikki says they spent five years going through Artificial Insemination and In Vitro Fertilization when God sent an unexpected adoption there way. Her aunt died suddenly leaving a five-year-old daughter, Amber, homeless (her birth father was incarcerated). *"The night I received the call from my father, I told him right then, 'Dad, I don't know what the family plans for Amber, but I feel we have to take her. I need to talk to Jason about it, but it just feels to me that this is God's Will.' In the background Jason was telling me, 'We don't need to talk about it— it's already decided.'"*

Nikki and Jason became parents in a matter of three days. *"Needless to say, that weekend Jason and I did a lot of talking, crying, praying and praising our Lord. His Will was being revealed to us in quite a HUGE and very deliberate way and there was no denying it. It was finally clear why we had undergone so many failed atempts at getting pregnant. God was preparing us for this moment,"* explained Nikki.

She adds, *"It was for one reason and one reason only we had to endure our trials and why Amber was taken out of her unhealthy environment and put into our home – it was God's purpose. We were designed and created to raise **this** child, and we are the couple chosen to guide her in God's plan for her own life. God chose **us** for this task and I am so extemely humbled that He would choose **me** to be her new mother.*

God does have a plan for each of us and there are times when we don't understand or even like it. Proverbs 19:21 says: 'Many are the plans in a man's heart, but it is the Lord's purpose that prevails.' Our lives are not about going through life doing what pleases us and experiencing the 'normal' American life. Our lives are not even about us at all. It's about fulfilling the puspose God has for each of us," Nikki concluded.

Blessings in Disguise

So, what are the blessings of barrenness? Growing in faith and obedience are the first blessings that come to my mind. Be sure to continually use the "keys" I gave you in Chapter 2 – verses out of the Book of James that put

God's intentions into perspective. This time I am sharing *The Living Bible* version which I really enjoy: *"Dear brothers, is your life full of difficulties and temptations? Then be happy, for when the way is rough, your patience has a chance to grow. So let it grow, and don't try to squirm out of your problems. For when your patience is finally in full bloom, then you will be ready for anything, strong in character, full and complete."* (1:2-4)

During difficult times to come, remind yourself of God's love poured out for you in the verses listed in Chapter 4. He loves you so much that He sent His "only begotten Son" to earth to experience the emotions and dealings of human beings. For example, Jesus sees your sadness, He experienced it too when He faced sadness here on earth. He appreciates your loneliness; He experienced it too. He views the testing of your faith and He relates. His extreme faith was demonstrated on the cross. He was tested by the evil one just like you, and He overcame the temptation to sin. He knows the grief you experience through the loss of a child. His Father gave Him up for you. His love for you is immeasurable!

Another example of His protective love is in the form of the Holy Spirit whom He left to encourage and guide you. Call upon Him often; He will be there for you through thick and thin. He will aid you in making good decisions. He will lead you down the path of incredible blessings. And, as illustrated in Christine's testimony, He will eventually make you aware of why He chose this trial for you and how you are better for it. Continue to ask Him to speak to you and ask Him to make His wisdom clear to you.

Perhaps He'll make you more aware of the blessings in your life like He did with my friend, Cindi McMennamin. After experiencing secondary infertility He showed her how to focus on what she had instead of what was missing in her life. Cindi told me she was confused, and a little bit scared. She couldn't figure out why God would withhold another baby from her and her husband. She wondered if He wasn't pleased with the way that she had parented her daughter.

It had been two years since Cindi and her husband decided they wanted another child, yet nothing was happening. She said that getting pregnant with her daughter had been so easy, so she couldn't imagine what the problem was. The months passed and the McMennamins prayed fervently for a second child. They decided to undergo tests for secondary infertility. Finally, the doctor called Cindi with the news. He told her that the miracle baby she had been praying for had been born three years earlier. The doctor explained that there was fertility incompatibility between Cindi and her husband and

CHAPTER 11—FEELING DESPERATE FOR GOD

medically speaking, they shouldn't have been able to have any children at all!

Cindi says that as she hung up the phone, she sank to her knees in gratitude to the Lord. By concentrating so fully on what she didn't have, she realized she had lost focus of the blessing she already had—a happy, healthy three-year-old, whom she had almost taken for granted.[2]

God is so good. He enhanced Karen's relationship with her loved ones through this trial: *"If there is a good side to infertility, it is that infertility has brought me closer to God. Despite the difficult times my husband and I have lived through, our love has grown stronger. Secondary infertility also has made me even more grateful for our daughter. I never take a moment of our lives together for granted."*[3]

Some of you will learn the importance of surrender through this trial. For instance, Patty surrendered her inability to conceive and "the ache" was removed thereafter: *"I understand those who ache to give birth to a child. I was once that way, but I never became pregnant. A few years ago, through our church, we were involved in a camp for foster children. As a result of our camp experience, we became interested in helping children who needed foster care.*

During the past two years, we have had 12 children pass through our home. There were a few we fell in love with, but they either went home or to a relative's house. We were okay with that, because we wanted what was best for the children.

Currently we have a foster child who has stolen our hearts. If the parents' rights are terminated, we plan to adopt her. Through this process, our ache for a birth child has diminished. Through the process of being a foster parent, God is changing dreams for the type of child who will satisfy our desire."[4]

God may be steering your life in a different direction than you planned like He did with Nikki. She and her husband are still experiencing peaks and valleys as they try to provide Amber with a brother or sister. *"While my trial of infertility is still ongoing, I am thankful for the strength, faith, and endurance God has blessed me with. I have cried out to Him more, leaned on Him more, trusted Him more, prayed more, desired Him more, and even loved Him more because of all the work He has done in my life and that He continues to do.*

I see the impact this trial has had on my family and friends and I know they see God in all of it – that is awesome to me. What an amazing harvest I get to be a laborer in. I pray that your life will be changed drastically through your trial – it will be if you let God do what He does best—be God." Nikki advised.

Through God's Word you've learned to rely on Him and perhaps you needed to learn to allow others to bear your burden as well. You may need to let down your protective walls and allow carefully selected people to ride out the storm with you. Many of the ladies in this book referred to their support groups being key components in their healing. I admire them for allowing me to include their photos for you. When you feel there's no end in sight, go back and look at these beautiful families and remind yourself that their storm eventually came to an end and so will yours.

Perhaps God will use this trial to help you appreciate the child He will soon bless you with to a greater degree (remember the story I shared about my son)? Whatever your circumstances, I believe it is no coincidence that you discovered this book—it was divine intervention. God wants you to know He hasn't forgotten you. He loves you! Hopefully you can see this trial as a way to become desperate for Him, instead of wanting to run away from it or avoid it.

My prayer is that each one of you will search deep, deep in your hearts until you come to a point in your life when you can honestly say that you welcome what God has in store for you NO MATTER what it is. He may lead you to take a break from the testing to solidify your marriage. He may send adoption or foster care your way, or He may direct you to continue living as a complete family.

Then you will be able to thank God for this trial and be grateful for his loving care like Sheri is: *"There comes a point when all you can do is run to the arms of Jesus. He's there seeing every single tear and feeling every single pain. It's not in vain—He has a perfect plan. He is using infertility to make you into the woman he wants you to be – the woman He can use for His ways and His glory. He's growing you. He's making you better and stronger—more like Him. He suffered, so you will suffer. It's for something greater than you can see at this present time. It's perfect."*

So, what will your "story" include? Surrender... a renewed satisfaction with your life... a purpose for living? How will this trial culminate for you in regard to your walk with the Lord? Whatever the outcome your journey includes, you can be assured that through a deeper relationship with Christ, stronger faith, and the return of joy and peace in your life, God will use the trial of infertility as a *blessing in disguise!*

CHAPTER 11—FEELING DESPERATE FOR GOD

It's in the Valleys I Grow

I have so much to learn
And my growth is very slow,
Sometimes I need the mountaintops,
But it's in the valleys I grow.

I do not always understand
Why things happen as they do,
But I am very sure of one thing.
My Lord will see me through.

My little valleys are nothing
When I picture Christ on the cross.
He went through the valley of death;
His victory was Satan's loss.
Forgive me, Lord, for complaining
When I'm feeling so very low.
Just give me a gentle reminder
That it's in the valleys I grow.

Continue to strengthen me. Lord,
And use my life each day
To share your love with others
And help them find their way.
Thank you for valleys. Lord,
For this one thing I know:
The mountaintops are glorious
But it's in the valleys I grow!

An excerpt from a poem by Jane Eggleston[5]

"The steps of good men are directed by the Lord. He delights in each step they take. If they fall it isn't fatal, for the Lord holds them with his hand." **Psalm 37:23-24 (NLT)**

Notes

Introduction

1. 1 Corinthians 2:9—*"However, as it is written: 'No eye has seen, no ear has heard, no mind has conceived what God has prepared for those who love him.'"*
2. Ephesians 1:4-5—*"For he chose us in him before the creation of the world to be holy and blameless in his sight. In love he predestined us to be adopted as his sons through Jesus Christ, in accordance with his pleasure and will…"*

Chapter 2

1. Philippians 4:7
2. Excerpts taken from "More than Enough," an article by Christy Harker, in *Stepping Stones* newsletter, C/O Bethany Christian Services, Oct./Nov. 2002.
3. Thomas Mercer, Senior Pastor, High Desert Church, Victorville, CA 92394.

Chapter 3

1. Hannah's story is found in 1 Samuel 1:1-28.
2. *The Living Bible*, page 403, a paraphrase of verse 1:18.
3. Copyright © 1983 by Houghton Mifflin Company. Adapted and reproduced by permission from *The American Heritage Dictionary, Office Edition*, page 285.
4. Published by Bethany Christian Services, www.bethany.org. Quote taken from article titled, "Infertility Awareness Week" in the Aug./Sept. 2000 issue of *Stepping Stones*.
5. Matthew 14:13—*"When Jesus heard what had happened, he withdrew by boat privately to a solitary place."*
6. Matthew 14:23—*"After he had dismissed them, he went up on a mountainside by himself to pray, when evening came, he was there alone…"*
7. Hebrews 13:5
8. 2 Peter 3:9—*"The Lord is not slow in keeping his promise, as some understand slowness. He is patient with you, not wanting anyone to perish, but everyone to come to repentance."*

9. John 10:10— *"The thief comes only to seal and kill and destroy; I have come that they may have life, and have it to the full."*
10. Matthew 15:8-9—*"These people honor me with their lips, but their hearts are far from me. They worship me in vain; their teachings are but rules taught by men."*
11. Colossians 2:20-23— *"Since you died with Christ to the basic principles of this world, why, as though you still belonged to it, do you submit to its rules?' Do not handle! Do not taste! Do not touch!' These are all destined to perish with use, because they are based on human commands and teachings. Such regulations indeed have an appearance of wisdom, with their self-imposed worship, their false humility and their harsh treatment of the body, but they lack any value in restraining sensual indulgence."*
12. Luke 15:24—*"For this son of mine was dead and alive again; he was lost and is found."*

Chapter 4

1. Rebekah's story is found in Genesis 24:1-67 and 25:19-26.
2. 1 Corinthians 2:9—*"However, as it is written: 'No eye has seen, no ear has heard, no mind has conceived what God has prepared for those who love him.'"*
3. "I Go Not to the 'Yes,' but to the 'No'" an article by Elizabeth Price, published in *Stepping Stones* newsletter, Aug./Sept. 2002.
4. Matthew 6:9-13—*"This, then, is how you should pray: 'Our Father in heaven, hallowed by your name, your kingdom come, your will be done on earth as it is in heaven. Give us today our daily bread. Forgive us our debts, as we also have forgiven our debtors. And lead us not into temptation, but deliver us from the evil one.'"*
5. Quote by John Van Regenmortar, *Stepping Stones* newsletter, Jan./Feb. 2003 issue, article titled, "The Questions are Endless."
6. Dr. Earl W. (Sandy) Stradtman, M.D., P.C., author of the article "He Didn't Give Me Answers, He Gave Me Himself," printed in *Stepping Stones* newsletter, Feb./March 2001.

Chapter 5

1. Sarah's story begins in Genesis 15:1.
2. 2 Corinthians 2:11—*"In order that Satan might not outwit us. For we are not unaware of his schemes."*

3. Definition taken from *The American Heritage Dictionary*, page 274.
4. IBID, page 674.
5. IBID, page 80.
6. Isaiah 14:12-15—*"How you are fallen from heaven, O Lucifer, son of the morning! How you are cut down to the ground – mighty though you were against the nations of the world. For you said to yourself, 'I will ascend to heaven and rule the angels. I will take the highest throne. I will preside on the Mount of Assembly far away in the north. I will climb to the highest heavens and be like the Most High.' But instead, you will be brought down to the pit of hell, down to its lowest depths."*
7. Ephesians 6:12—*"For we are not fighting against people made of flesh and blood, but against persons without bodies – the evil rulers of the unseen world, those mighty satanic beings and great evil princes of darkness who rule this world; and against huge numbers of wicked spirits in the spirit world."*
8. List taken from page 1466 of *The Living Bible*.
9. 2 Corinthians 10:3-5—*"For though we live in the world, we do not wage war as the world does. The weapons we fight with are not the weapons of the world. On the contrary, they have divine power to demolish strongholds. We demolish arguments and every pretension that sets itself up against the knowledge of God, and we take captive every thought to make it obedient to Christ."*
10. "Seven Reasons Not to Worry" taken from page 1338 of *The Living Bible*.
11. Paraphrase of verse 6:25 on page 1338 of *The Living Bible*.
12. Paraphrase of verse 6:34 on page 1338 of *The Living Bible*.
13. Pastor Mercer's sermon was given as part of a nationwide "40 Days of Purpose" campaign. Pastor Mercer gave the following credit: *"A special word of thanks to Pastor Rick Warren and the Saddleback Church in Lake Forest, CA. Pastor Rick's vision and material formed the basis for much of the content in these seven presentations [40 Days of Purpose]. HDC [High Desert Church] participated with thousands of churches around the world during October and November, 2003, for the FdoP campaign. Many of our people will never be the same."*
14. Paraphrase of Isaiah 59:1-2 on page 1044 of *The Living Bible*.
15. "Divine Surrender" Bible Study, by Lorie Coleman, Freedom Ministries, Apple Valley, CA.
16. As defined in *The American Heritage Dictionary*, page 343.

17. Definition taken from *The American Heritage Dictionary*, page 544.
18. Beth Moore, author of the Bible study "Breaking Free," *Making Liberty in Christ a Reality in Life,* LifeWay Press, Nashville, TN, 2002, page 58. Used with permission.
19. Definitions from *The American Heritage Dictionary,* page 642.
20. Poem printed in *Stepping Stones* newsletter, July/Aug. 2004 edition.

Chapter 6

1. Elizabeth's story is found in Luke 1:1.
2. *On Death and Dying* published by Touchstone Books, 1997, ISBN 0-684-84223-8.
3. Quotes taken from Lisa DeSherlia, author of the article "Secondary Infertility: A Prayer," printed in the Jan./Feb. 2003 *Stepping Stones* newsletter.
4. *The American Heritage Dictionary*, page599.
5. Mary Utzig, author of the article, "To Be a Mom," printed in *Stepping Stones* newsletter, Aug./Sept. 2002 issue.
6. *The American Heritage Dictionary*, page72.
7. "A Woman's Heart, God's Dwelling Place," a Bible study by Beth Moore, LifeWay Press, Nashville, TN, page 36. Used with permission.
8. Poem printed in *Stepping Stones* newsletter, Aug./Sept 2000 issue.

Chapter 7

1. Manoah's wife's story begins in Judges 13:1.
2. Paraphrase of Judges 13:5 found on page 375 of *The Living Bible*.
3. Page 955 of *The Living Bible*.
4. Proverbs 31:31 paraphrase on page 961 of *The Living Bible*.
5. Quote by Dixie Lewis, author of "Healing Moments" article in the Dec. 2000/Jan. 2001 *Stepping Stones* newsletter.

Chapter 8

1. Rachel's story can be found in the Book of Genesis from 29:1 to 35:19.
2. Description of Rachel on page 59 of *The Living Bible*.
3. *The Living Bible* paraphrase for verses 4:8 on page 1922.
4. From WHAT TO EXPECT WHEN YOU'RE EXPERIENCING INFERTILITY by Debby Peoples and Harriette Rovner Ferguson. Copyright

1998 by Debby Peoples and Harriette Rovner Ferguson. Used by permission of W.W. Norton & Company, Inc. Page 137.
5. *When Empty Arms Become a Burden* by Sandra Glahn and William Cutrer, M.D., published by Broadman & Holman Publishers, page 105. Used by permission.
6. Excerpts taken from "Coping with Christmas" article by Debbie Lute. Printed in the *Stepping Stones* Dec. 2001/Jan. 2002 issue.
7. Psalm 66:10 – "For you, O God, tested us; you refined us like silver."
8. Daniel 12:10a – "Many will be purified, made spotless and refined, but the wicked will continue to be wicked."
9. *Stepping Stones* newsletter, Dec. 2002 issue.
10. *Stepping Stones* newsletter, Dec. 2001/Jan. 2002 issue.
11. Printed in the June/July 2001 edition of *Stepping Stones* newsletter.
12. Article titled "Help Wanted."
13. "The Day I Turned Back," by Allison MacPhail, *Stepping Stones*, June/July 2001 issue.
14. Poem printed in the Dec. 2001/Jan. 2002 *Stepping Stones* newsletter.

Chapter 9

1. Article printed in the Oct./Nov. 2002 edition of *Stepping Stones* newsletter.
2. Excerpts taken from the article, "Old Dead Twig," written by Ruth Leamy and printed in the Sept./Oct. 2003 issue of *Stepping Stones* newsletter.
3. Poem printed in the Jan./Feb. 2003 issue of *Stepping Stones* newsletter.
4. Kathleen A. Massey, author of "Careless Words," an article printed in the Sept/Oct. 2003 issue of *Stepping Stones* newsletter.
5. "After My Miscarriage…"by Lorena Brant, *Stepping Stones* newsletter, April/May 2001 issue.
6. Terry Willits, author of "How to Encourage an Infertile Friend" published in the *Stepping Stones* newsletter, Aug./Sept. 2000 issue.
7. Quote taken from "My Sister Sent Me Flowers: Experiencing Sensitivity in an Insensitive World" by Angie Curlette printed in the Aug./Sept. 2000 *Stepping Stones* newsletter.
8. Quote taken from Barbara Fletcher, author of "An Awesome Privilege" printed in the Oct./Nov. 2001 issue of *Stepping Stones* newsletter.
9. "A Road Less Traveled" by Janet Fasnacht, printed in the Feb./March 2001 *Stepping Stones* newsletter.

Chapter 10

1. IBID, pages 57 to 68.
2. Poem printed in the *Stepping Stones* newsletter, Jan./Feb. 2003 issue.
3. Quote from Karen (last name not given) in the article, "Living Positively Without Children," by John and Sylvia Van Regenmorter and printed in the *Stepping Stones* newsletter, Feb./March 2002.
4. Page 1807 – paraphrase of Ephesians 1:8, in *The Living Bible*.
5. Quotes taken from Dixie Lewis, author of "Healing Moments," an article in the Dec. 2000/Jan. 2001 *Stepping Stones* newsletter.
6. Poem printed in the *Stepping Stones* newsletter, May/June 2003.
7. IBID, pages 44-46.
8. *The Living Bible* page 9.
9. Article by Roxanne Griswold printed in the May/June 2003 issue of *Stepping Stones* newsletter.
10. Quotes from Tammy Anderson's article, "Is there Only ONE Happy Ending?" *Stepping Stones* newsletter, Feb/March 2002.
11. Quotes from John and Sylvia Van Regenmorter in their article titled, "Living Positively Without Children," printed in the Feb./March 2002 issue of *Stepping Stones* newsletter.

Chapter 11

1. Taken from *Purpose-Driven Life, The* by RICK WARREN. Copyright 2002 by Rick Warren. Used by permission of The Zondervan Corporation, page 20.
2. This story, by Cindi McMenamin, first appeared in "Treasures of a Woman's Heart," compiled by Lynn D. Morrissey, Starburst Publishers, 2000, pg. 249. Used by permission.
3. Quote from Karen Lally—"Seeking Resolution," *Stepping Stones* newsletter, Dec. 2000/ Jan. 2001.
4. Quotes from Patty Bye, author of "God Changed Our Hopes and Dreams," printed in the Aug./Sept. 2002 issue of *Stepping Stones* newsletter.
5. An excerpt from a poem by Jane Eggleston. To read the entire poem, visit www.alltel.net-cbmpaul/thought.htm. Printed in the Feb./March 2002 issue of *Stepping Stones* newsletter.

Appendix A
Resources

Note from the Author: I have not personally read all of these books or investigated all of the resources, nor do I know if they are all Christian-based. However, I feel reading about the subject you are dealing with aids you in understanding, overcoming and accepting obstacles and issues involved. An asterisk denotes the resources I am familiar with.

INFERTILITY Books:

A Hope Deferred
By Jill Baughan

BioBasic Series: Basic Questions on Sexuality and Reproductive Technology
By Various Authors Associated with The Center for Bioethics and Human Dignity Kregel Publications, 1998

Coping with Infertility
By Judith A. Stigger

Cradle of Dreams
By Joseph Bentz, Bethany House, 2001

Dear God, Why Can't We Have a Baby?
By John and Sylvia Van Regenmorter and Joe S. McIlhaney, Jr. M.D.

Empty Womb, Aching Heart
Marlo Schalesky
Bethany House, 2001

From Infertility to In Vitro Fertilization
By Geoffrey Sher, M.D. and Virginia A. Marriage R.N., M.N.

Give Us a Child
By Lynda Stephenson

Infertility: Finding God's Peace in the Journey
By Lois Flowers, Harvest House © 2003.

Infertility on the Internet: How to Get On-Line and In Charge of Your Fertility
By Julie Watson, Conceiving Concepts, 1997

Lethal Secrets: The Shocking Consequences and Unsolved Problems of Artificial Insemination
By Annette Baran and Reuben Pannor

Living with Infertility: Christian Support Studies for Individuals or Groups
By Roger and Robin Sonnenberg, Concordia Publishing House, 1994

Moments for Couples Who Long for Children
By Ginger Garrett
Navpress, Copyright © 2003

Overcoming Infertility
By Robert Nachtigall, M.D. and Elizabeth Mehren

Rain Dance
By Joy E. DeKok, Pleasant Word, ©2003

* *Taking Charge of Your Fertility*
By Toni Weschler, MPH, HarperCollins Publishers, Inc., 1995

Taste of Tears, Touch of God
By Ann Kiemel Anderson

* *The Ache for a Child*
By Debra Bridwell, Micra Communications, 1999
(Originally published in 1994 by Victor Books)

The Infertility Book: A Comprehensive Medical & Emotional Guide
By Carla Harkness

The Long Awaited Child
By Tracie Peterson
Bethany House, 2001

The Long-Awaited Stork: A Guide to Parenting after Infertility
By Ellen Glazer

Water from the Rock
Finding God's Comfort in the Midst of Infertility
By Donna Gibbs, Becky Garrett, Phyllis Rabon, Moody Press 2002

* *What to Expect When You're Experiencing Infertility*
By Debby Peoples and Harriette Rovner Ferguson, C.S.W.

* *When Empty Arms Became a Heavy Burden*
By Sandra Glahn and William Cutrer, M.D., Broadman & Holman Publishers, 1997

When a Husband is Infertile
By Byron C. Calhoun, Baker books, 1994

When the Cradle is Empty: Answering Tough Questions About Infertility
By John and Sylvia Van Regenmorter
Focus on the Family and Tyndale Publishing House, Copyright © 2004

INFERTILITY Newsletters:

* Resolve
617-623-1156

* Stepping Stones
1-800-BETHANY or www.bethany.org

SECONDARY INFERTILITY Books:

One Child by Choice
By Sharryl Hawke and David Knox

Wanting Another Child
By Harriet Fishman Simons, Lexington Books, 1995

MOVING ON AS A COMPLETE FAMILY Books:

Childless is Not Less
By Vicky Love

Sweet Grapes: How to Stop Being Infertile and Start Living Again
By Jean W. Carter, M.D. and Michael Carter, Ph.D.

MOVING ON AS A COMPLETE FAMILY Resource:

Childfree Network – 916-773-7178
A national organization that provides education, support, and resources for child-free individuals and couples.

INFERTILITY Support Groups:

Bethany Christian Services, Stepping Stones – Go to www.bethany.org/step to access their support group directory. The data includes contact information, meeting times, purpose, etc.

RESOLVE – Go to www.resolve.org to access their list of 50 chapters. According to the website, the volunteer-run chapters offer many services to members including local educational meetings, help lines, support groups and conferences.

INFERTILITY Resources:

American Board of Medical Specialties (ABMS)—This website allows you to verify the board certification, status, and location of physicians certified by one or more of the 24 member boards of the ABMS. certifieddoctor.org

American Infertility Association—A national organization dedicated to assisting those facing reproductive health issues, americaninfertility.org

American Society for Reproductive Medicine—An organization devoted to advancing knowledge and expertise in reproductive medicine and biology, asrm.org

Christian Counseling

The following organizations may be able to help you find a Christian counselor in your area:

American Association of Christian Counselors (AACC) aacc.net
Christian Association of Psychological Studies (CAPS) caps. net

The Endometriosis Association, 800-922-ENDO

Offers support to women with endometriosis, including a newsletter, video and audiotapes, support groups, and a help line.

Ferre Institute, Inc., 315-724-4348

Offers brochures, a newsletter, and a lending library of books related to infertility.

Hannah's Prayer—Hannah's Prayer provides Christian support for infertility challenges including infertility or the loss of a child any time from conception through early infancy. Hannah's Prayer also offers an email and Internet support group, hannah.org

Infertility Awareness Association of Canada—IAAC provides educational material, support, and assistance to those experiencing the medical, emotional, and financial effects of infertility, iaac.ca

Inciid—This organization, pronounced "Inside," offers a wealth of medical information, statistics, and resources on infertility. It also provides a state-by-state listing of specialists, including reproductive endocrinologist. inciid.org

National Infertility Network Exchange, 516-794-5772

Offers national support for infertility and adoption, including referrals and a newsletter.

* Resolve—A national infertility organization with a nationwide network of chapters. Resolve provides education, advocacy, and support, resolve.org

Stepping Stones Discussion Forums—The participants of the forums are invited to post questions, share experiences, and offer helpful information and encouragement, stepforums.bethany.org

Women's Health Connection – 800-366-6632
A consumer health education resource network dedicated to educating women about hormone-related disorders such as PMS, menopause, infertility, and postpartum depression. Publishes a newsletter that highlights articles on current women's health topics and hormone disorders.

GRIEVING Books:

Disappointment with God
By Philip Yancy

Don't Take My Grief Away
By Doug Manning

Life After Loss
By Bob Deits

PREGNANCY LOSS Books:

Empty Arms: Emotional Support for Those who Have Suffered Miscarriage or Stillbirth
By Pam Vredevelt, Multnomah Books, 1995

From Sorrow to Serenity
By Susan Fletcher, Hunter House Publications, 1998

Good Mourning
By Judy Morrow and Nancy DeHamer

I Can't Find a Heartbeat
By Melissa Sexson Hanson
Review and Herald Publishing Co., 1999

*In Heavenly Arms—Grieving the Loss, Healing the Wounds of Miscarriage
By Shari L. Bridgman, Ph.D.

Morning Will Come
By Sandy Day
Caleb Cares, Copyright © 1993

No New Baby
By Marilyn Gryte

Preventing Miscarriage: The Good News
By Jonathon Scher, M.D. and Carol Dix

Surviving Pregnancy Loss
By Rochelle Friedman, M.D.

Threads of Hope, Pieces of Joy: A Pregnancy Loss Bible Study for Group or Individual Use
By Teale Fackler and Gwen Kik
Benjamin Books (1999)

When a Baby Dies
By Ronald H. Nash, Zondervan, 1999

When Pregnancy Fails: Families Coping with Miscarriage, Stillbirth and Infant Death
By Susan Borg and Judith Lasker

PREGNANCY LOSS Newsletters:

Bereaved Parents Share II, free, quarterly newsletter
Write to: Ceci Kent, PO Box 121, Centralia, WA 98531

M.E.N.D.—Mommies Enduring Neonatal Death, bimonthly newsletter
Call 888.695.MEND or visit www.mend.org

Nathaniel's Friends, bimonthly, donation-based newsletter
Write to: bayonne@bigvalley.net

PREGNANCY LOSS Support Groups:

Puzzle Peace Infertility/pregnancy loss, Christ-centered support group in Hudsonville, MI
Call Martheen at 616.224.7488 or write to step@bethany.org

PREGNANCY LOSS Resources:

Caleb Ministries—A Christian ministry offering help for women who have experienced infertility, miscarriage, stillbirth, early infant death, or are post-abortive, calebministries.org

Centering Corporation, 402-553-1200
Offers a catalog of books on miscarriage, stillbirth and grief.

CLIMB—Center for Loss in Multiple Births – 907-746-6123
Publishes quarterly newsletter and contact list for parents who have lost one or more babies.

Compassionate Friends
PO Box 3696, Oak Brook, IL 60522-3696, (708) 990-0010
A nationwide, self-help group offering support for those mourning the death of a child, including by miscarriage or stillbirth. Also offers local chapter monthly meetings, books, and a quarterly newsletter.

H.A.N.D. of Santa Clara County
PO Box 341, Los Gatos, CA 95031, (408) 732-3228
H.A.N.D. (Helping After Neonatal Death) offers support to parents during the normal mourning following a childbearing loss. Offers phone peer counseling, a newsletter, a resource library, grief support groups within California, and assistance in starting support groups elsewhere. It also offers in-service workshops for medical professionals.

Mommies Enduring Neonatal Death—A Christian non-profit organization that reaches out to those who have lost a child to miscarriage, stillbirth, or infant death, mend.org

Pregnancy and Infant Loss Center
1421 E. Wayzata Blvd., #30 Wayzata, MN 55391 (612) 473-9372
Offers the Loving Arms newsletter, referrals to support groups, and information for related areas such as funeral options, high-risk pregnancy, and surviving siblings.

SHARE: Pregnancy and Infant Loss Support, Inc.
St. Joseph Health Center, 300 First Capitol Drive, St. Charles, MO 63301-2893, (314) 947-6164
Offers emotional, physical, spiritual, and social support for those who are troubled by the tragic death of a baby through miscarriage, stillbirth, or newborn death. The support includes a bimonthly newsletter, and 250 chapters internationally. Also provides education about bereaved parents.

UNITE, Inc. Grief Support
C/0 Jeanes Hospital, 7600 Central Avenue, Philadelphia, PA 19111-2499, (215) 728-3777
This is a national grief support for those who have experienced pregnancy loss. Offers a quarterly newsletter and referrals to local support groups.

ADOPTION Books:

* *"A" is for Adoption Booklet*
Bethany Christian Services

* *Adoption as a Ministry, Adoption as a Blessing*
By Michelle Gardner, Copyright © 2003
Pleasant Word, a Division of Winepress Publishing

* *Adoption without Fear*
Edited by James L. Gritter, M.S.W.
Corona Publishing Company, San Antonio, TX, Copyright © 1989

Adopting After Infertility
By Patricia Irwin Johnston
Perspectives Press, 1992

Adopting the Older Child
By Claudia L. Jewett

Being Adopted, The Lifelong Search for Self
By David M. Brodzinsky, Ph.D., Marshall D. Schechter, M.D. and Robin Marantz Henig

* *Chosen Families*
By Kay Marshall Strom
Pyranee Books, Published by Zondervan Publishing House, Grand Rapids, MI, Copyright © 1985

Financing Adoption, free information packet
Call 1.800.613.3188 or visit nab@bethany.org

* *How it Feels to be Adopted*
By Jill Krementz

Loved by Choice: True Stories that Celebrate Adoption
By Susan Horner & Kelly Fordyce Martindale, Revell, Grand Rapids, MI, ©2002

Open Adoption: My Story of Love and Laughter
By Ann Kiemel Anderson

Raising Adopted Children
By Lois Melina

Should You Adopt?
By Christine Moriarty Field
Fleming H. Revell, 1997

* *The Missing Piece*
By Lee Ezell

ADOPTION Resources:

Adopted Child
PO Box 9362, Moscow, ID 83843, (208) 882-1794
Offers educational material for adoptive parenting.

Adoptive Families of America (AFA)
3333 Highway 100 North Minneapolis, MN 55422-2752 (800) 372-3300
www.adopting.org
The largest national adoptive family non-profit support organization (20,000 members). AFA offers adoptive parent support, a magazine, a conference and a book catalog.

* America World Adoption Association
888-ONE-CHILD, www.awaa.org
AWAA is committed to helping America's families and the world's orphans experience the love of God in Jesus through the "Spirit of Adoption."

American Academy of Adoption Attorneys – 202-832-2222
A national organization of attorneys who practice or have otherwise distinguished themselves in the field of adoption law.

American Adoption Congress (AAC)
1000 Connecticut Avenue, N.W., Suite 9, Washington, D.C. 20036, (202) 483-3399
Umbrella organization for reform movement; conferences, newsletter, referrals

* Bethany Christian Services
901 Eastern Avenue, N.E., PO Box 294, Grand Rapids, MI 49501-0294
1-800-BETHANY, info@bethany.org
Bethany is a not-for profit, pro-life, Christian adoption and family services agency with more than 75 locations in 30 states and ministries in 15 other countries.

Child Welfare League of America (CWLA)
440 First Street, NW, Suite 310, Washington, DC 20001-2085
(202) 638-2952 Fax (202) 638-4004
Adoptive and foster parenting concerns, books, setting of public policy.

Council for Equal Rights In Adoption (CERA)
401 East 74th Street, Suite 17D
New York, NY 10021-3919, (212) 988-0110
Adoption reform, search and support group referrals, newsletter and a conference.

* Dave Thomas Foundation for Adoption – 614-764-8454

* Eastern Europe Adoption Coalition
www.eeadopt.org

Families for Private Adoption – 202-722-0338
Supports and educates families who are interested in private, non-agency adoption. Helps families to network with other adoptive families as well as other adoption organizations.

* Holt International Children's Services
PO Box 2880 Eugene, OR 97402 (503) 687-2202
A Christian International Adoption Agency, also offers a bi-monthly magazine.

Jewell Among Jewels Adoption Network, Inc.
www. adoptionjewels.org
Through writing and speaking, Jewell Among Jewels seek; to honor, educate, and encourage those touched by adoption,

* KidSave International
1-888-KID-SAVE, info@kidsave.org
Kidsave works on a year-round basis to expand he use of summer camp programs as a method used by adoption agencies to place older children regardless of country of origin.

National Adoption Center (not an agency) – 215-735-9988
An organization devoted to helping children with special needs and from minority cultures to find loving homes.

National Committee for Adoption, Inc.
1933-17th Street, NW Washington, D.C. 20009-6207 (202) 328-1200
Offers information for those seeking to adopt.

* Nightlight Christian Adoptions
801 E. Chapman Avenue, Suite 106, Fullerton, CA 92831
714-278-1020, www.nightlight.org

Nightlight is a non-profit adoption agency licensed by the State of California to provide adoption services.

North American Council on Adoptable Children (NACAC)
970 Raymond Avenue, Suite 106, St. Paul, MN 55114-1149
(612) 644-3036 Fax (612) 644-9848
Adoptive family support, special needs adoption, education and a conference.

* Olive Crest Foster Family and Adoption Agency
1-800-550-CHILD, 1-800-74-FOSTER, www.olivecrest.org
Olive Crest operates 20 residential homes, foster family and adoption agencies, and children's centers for high-risk youth.

Pact-An Adoption Alliance
3315 Sacramento Street, Suite #239, San Francisco, CA 94118,
(415) 221-6957
Facilitates low fee adoptions for infants of color, including trans-racial adoptions.

* RESOLVE
617-623-1156, www.resolve.org
A large, national organization with local chapters offering compassionate and informed support related to infertility, miscarriage or adoption. Offers a support line, quarterly newsletters, symposiums and workshops, pre-adoption meetings, and a lending library.

Appendix B

Note from the author: The following questionnaire, evaluation, and Biblical list of spiritual gifts are tools the pastors at my home church use to help members determine what their spiritual gifts are. The author and/or origin of these tools are unknown.

Spiritual Gifts Questionnaire

In answering these questions, place the appropriate numerical value on the line next to each question depending on which response is true for you.

MUCH = 3
SOME = 2
LITTLE = 1
NOT AT ALL = 0

____ 1. Do you enjoy assisting leaders to relieve them for their particular job?
____ 2. When you hear of someone in the hospital, do you feel a desire to go and comfort him or her?
____ 3. Do you manage your money well in order to give generously to the Lord's work?
____ 4. Do you adapt easily to a different culture than your own?
____ 5. Are you burdened to meet non-Christians in order to win them to Christ?
____ 6. Are you single and enjoying it?
____ 7. Have you had the desire to care for the spiritual needs of a group of people.
____ 8. Are you effective in persuading others to move toward Biblical objectives?
____ 9. Do you almost always feel certain God will keep His promises in spite of external circumstances?
____ 10. Do you effectively apply Biblical truth to your own life?
____ 11. Have you often been able to encourage people to trust God in time of need?
____ 12. Do you feel a lot of compassion for those who are suffering physically, and do you think of ways to help them?
____ 13. Do you enjoy giving to the Lord's work without asking whether or not you can afford it right now?

_____ 14. Do you know where you are going, and see other Christians follow you?
_____ 15. Are you able to organize ideas, people, things, and time for more effective ministry?
_____ 16. Do you sense an unusual assurance from God that He will do the impossible to fulfill a special work?
_____ 17. Do you find it easy to organize your thoughts and explain them to people?
_____ 18. Do you find you are a good and patient listener?
_____ 19. Do you study and read a great deal in order to learn Biblical truth?
_____ 20. Do you accurately recognize whether a teaching is of God, of Satan, or of human origin?
_____ 21. Do you enjoy doing routine tasks that lead to more effective ministry by others?
_____ 22. Are you thrilled when someone asks you to help financially in some project, seeing this as a great honor or privilege?
_____ 23. Do you have a knack for making strangers feel comfortable in your home?
_____ 24. Do you relate well to Christians of different races, language, or cultures?
_____ 25. Do you find yourself regularly sharing the Gospel message with non-believers?
_____ 26. Do you enjoy taking care of physical tasks for the church?
_____ 27. Do you enjoy the responsibility for the spiritual well being of a group of Christians?
_____ 28. Are you able to make effective and efficient plans to accomplish goals of the group?
_____ 29. Does "in-depth" Bible study come easy for you?
_____ 30. Have others encouraged you to have a special ministry to the sick and suffering, or commented on your suitability for such a ministry?
_____ 31. Do you take unexpected guests in stride, without apology for how your house may look?
_____ 32. Do you find it natural to explain that Jesus Christ died for our sins, and then to see a positive response by your listeners?
_____ 33. Does your desire to serve the Lord overshadow thoughts of getting married?
_____ 34. When someone asks a favor of you do you feel grateful they asked you?
_____ 35. Have other people asked you to help them "get organized"?
_____ 36. Has God done miraculous works for you and others in response to your prayers?
_____ 37. Have you been effective in communicating Biblical truth to others

so that their lives change in knowledge, attitudes, or conduct?

____ 38. Do you enjoy encouraging people who are going through personal problems and trials to "hang in there"?

____ 39. Do you feel certain you understand people's motives?

____ 40. Would you be happy as a teacher's aide in a Bible class?

____ 41. Do you enjoy making your home available to those in the Lord's service for an extended period of time?

____ 42. Do you think often of people in other cultures who have never heard of Christ?

____ 43. Has sexual fulfillment generally been low on your priority list?

____ 44. Are you always looking for jobs to do and to get done?

____ 45. Do others follow you because you have expert knowledge, which contributes to the ministry of the church?

____ 46. Do you have a knack for working out solutions to complicated problems in life?

____ 47. When you hear a spiritual question, are you anxious both to find and give the answer?

____ 48. Has God used you to get lazy or back-slidden Christians moving in the right direction again?

____ 49. Are you able to distinguish key and important facts of Scripture?

____ 50. Do you see through a phony before others recognize his phoniness?

____ 51. Do you feel deeply moved when confronted with urgent financial needs In God's work?

____ 52. Do you share joyfully how you became a Christian in a way that is meaningful to non-Christians?

____ 53. Do you feel indifferent toward getting married?

____ 54. Are you able to see what needs to be done in a particular task in the Lord's work and then do it?

____ 55. Have you been able to help people who have wandered out of Christian fellowship to come back?

____ 56. Does planning come easily to you?

____ 57. Do you seem to believe God's promises to a greater degree than most Christians?

____ 58. Do suggestions you make for solving problems regularly prove to be right?

____ 59. Do you enjoy acquiring and mastering new facts and principles of Bible truth?

____ 60. Do you feel great satisfaction for having helped someone else to be successful?

____ 61. Are you patient when you spend time with someone who is suffering, rather than wanting to leave as soon as you can?

____ 62. Do you enjoy having new people in your home?

____ 63. Do you make friends easily with people from different cultures?

____ 64. Have you been able to "feed" needy Christians by showing them relevant passages in the Bible and praying with them?

____ 65. Do you usually think about what can be done in the future rather than what is being done right now?

____ 66. Are you able to apply truth from the Bible to the specific needs of the Body?

____ 68. Have other people ever told you that you ought to be teaching on a regular basis?

____ 69. Have you perceived accurately a person under satanic influence?

Note: Number 67 is missing from this evaluation.

Spiritual Gifts Evaluation

Name _____
Date _____

Add up the scores from the question numbers in each row placing the sum in the "total" column. List your top three gifts in the "gift" column.

					TOTAL	GIFT
Row A	26	34	44	54		
Row B	17	37	47	68		
Row C	11	18	38	48		
Row D	3	13	22	51		
Row E	8	14	45	65		
Row F	2	12	30	61		
Row G	10	46	58	66		
Row H	19	29	49	59		
Row I	9	16	36	57		
Row J	20	39	50	69		
Row K	1	21	40	60		
Row L	15	28	35	56		
Row M	5	25	32	52		
Row N	7	27	55	64		
Row O	6	33	43	53		
Row P	23	31	41	62		
Row Q	4	24	42	63		

Note: The capital letters in each of the above rows correspond to the spiritual gifts defined in the "Spiritual Gifts" Biblical list on the next page.

A. Service
B. Teaching
C. Exhortation
D. Giving
E. Leadership
F. Mercy
G. Wisdom
H. Knowledge
I. Faith
J. Discerning of Spirits
K. Helps
L. Administration
M. Evangelist
N. Pastor
O. Celibacy
P. Hospitality
Q. Missionary

Biblical List of Spiritual Gifts

This list (all but celibacy/ hospitality and missionary) is derived from three New Testament passages: Romans 12, I Corinthians 12 and Ephesians 4. Note, since none of the three primary lists are complete/ and the three of them together are not complete, it is reasonable to assume that there may be more than we have identified here. Some have felt that intercession (a special ability to remain faithful in prayer for long periods of time)/ martyrdom, voluntary poverty, and exorcism should be considered gifts. There may be others as well.

A. Service: The gift of service is the special ability that God gives to certain members of the body of Christ to identify the unmet needs involved in a task related to God's work, and to make use of available resources to meet those needs and help accomplish the desired goals (Romans 12:7).

B. Teaching: The gift of teaching is the special ability that God gives to certain members of the Body of Christ to communicate spiritual truth in such a way that others will learn (Romans 12:7, 28-29, Ephesians 4:11).

C. Exhortation: The gift of exhortation is the special ability that God gives to certain members of the body of Christ to minister words of comfort, consolation, encouragement and counsel in such a way that others feel helped and healed (Romans 12:8).

D. Giving: The gift of giving is the special ability that God gives to certain members of the body of Christ to contribute their material resources to the work of the Lord with extreme liberality and cheerfulness (Romans 12:8).

E. Leadership: The gift of leadership is the special ability that God gives to certain members of the body of Christ to set goals in accordance with God's purpose for the future and to communicate in such a way that others voluntarily and harmoniously work together to accomplish those goals for the glory of God (Romans 12:8).

F. Mercy: The gift of mercy is the special ability that God gives to certain members of the body of Christ to feel genuine empathy and compassion for individuals who suffer distressing physical, mental or emotional problems, and to translate that compassion into cheerfully-done deeds that reflect Christ's love and alleviate the suffering (Romans 12:8).

G. Wisdom: The gift of wisdom is the special ability that God gives to certain members of the body of Christ to receive insight into how given knowledge may best be applied to specific needs arising in the body of Christ (I Corinthians 12:8).

H. Knowledge: The gift of knowledge is the special ability that God gives to certain members of the body of Christ to discover, accumulate, analyze and clarify spiritual truth (I Corinthians 12:8).

I. Faith: The gift of faith is the special ability that God gives to certain members of the body of Christ to discern with extraordinary confidence the will and purposes of God for the future of His work (I Corinthians 12:9).

J. Discerning the spirits: The gift of discerning of spirits is the special ability that God gives to certain members of the body of Christ to know with assurance whether certain behavior purported to be of God is in reality divine, human or satanic (I Corinthians 12:10).

K. Helps: The gift of helps is the special ability that God gives to certain members of the body of Christ to invest the talents they have in the life and ministry of other members of the body, thus helping others to increase the effectiveness of their spiritual gifts (I Corinthians 12:28).

L. Administration: The gift of administration is the special ability that God gives to certain members of the body of Christ to understand clearly the immediate and long-range goals of a particular part of the body of Christ and to devise and execute effective plans for the accomplishment of those goals (I Corinthians 12:28).

M. Evangelist: The gift of evangelist is the special ability that God gives to certain members of the body of Christ to share the gospel with unbelievers in such a way that men and women become Jesus' disciples and responsible members of the body of Christ on a regular

basis (Ephesians 4:11).

N. Pastor: The gift of pastor is the special ability that God gives to certain members of the body of Christ to assume a long-term personal responsibility for the spiritual welfare of a group of believers (Ephesians 4:11).

NOTE: You may possess the gift of pastor but never hold the New Testament office of pastor. Likewise, the specific duties of someone who holds the office will vary, depending on other gifts he may possess. For example, a man holding the office of pastor coupled with the gifts of leadership and administration may not want to spend much time preaching. In fact, unless God has gifted him so, it would be a disadvantage for him and the church. Likewise, a pastor who has the gift of teaching may spend less time evangelizing and administrating. The concept of a pastoral all-star who should spend his time doing everything is not only unbiblical, it doesn't work. When one understands the concept of spiritual gifts, a multiple-pastoral staff, with each pastor involved in different aspects of the church's ministry, has great credibility.

O. Celibacy: The gift of celibacy is the special ability that God gives to certain members of the body of Christ to remain single and satisfied, in order to more effectively serve Christ. (I Corinthians 7:7).

P. Hospitality: The gift of hospitality is the special ability that God gives to certain members of the body of Christ to provide open house and warm welcome for strangers in need of food and lodging (I Pete 4:9-10).

Q. Missionary: The gift of missionary is the special ability that God gives to certain members of the body of Christ to minister whatever other spiritual gifts they have in a second culture (Ephesians 3:6-7).

Note: The remaining gifts listed below have not been incorporated into the "Spiritual Gifts Questionnaire."

1. Prophecy: The gift of prophecy is the special ability that God gives to certain members of the body of Christ to boldly communicate c message of God to His people. (Romans 12:6, 1 Corinthians 12:10, 28-30 Ephesians 4:11).

2. Apostle: The gift of apostle is the special ability that God gives to certain members of the body of Christ to assume and exercise general leadership over a number of churches with an extraordinary authority in spiritual matters that is spontaneously recognized and appreciated b) those churches (I Corinthians 12:28-29, Ephesians 4:11).

NOTE: The gifts of prophecy and apostle described here have continued throughout church history. But they should not be confused with the offices of apostle and prophet, which were both foundational to the church and ended in the first century when God's revelation of the New Testament record was completed (I Corinthians 9:1, Ephesians 2:20, Revelation 21:14).

The remainder of the gifts listed here are commonly characterized as "sign gifts."

"They are not incorporated into the worship and programs here at High Desert Church simply because what seems to characterize their manifestations within today's Christian community does not fit the Biblical record.

1. Miracles: The gift of miracles is the special ability that God gives to certain members of the body of Christ to serve as human intermediaries through whom it pleases God to perform powerful acts that are perceived by observers to have altered the ordinary course ol nature (I Corinthians 12:10, 28-29).

2. Tongues: The gift of tongues is the special ability that God gives to certain members of the body of Christ to speak in a language they have never learned. (Acts 2:4,1 Corinthians 12:28-29).

3. Interpretation: The gift of interpretation is the special ability that God gives to certain members of the body of Christ to make known in the vernacular the message of one who speaks in tongues (I Corinthians 12:10, 30).

4. Healing: The gift of healing is the special ability that God gives to certain members of the body of Christ to serve as human intermediaries through whom it pleases God to cure illness and restore health apart from the use of natural means (I Corinthians 12:9, 28-30).

Appendix C
Answers to Fill-in-the Blank Verses:

CHAPTER 2

2 Chronicles 16:9a: *"For the eyes of the Lord range throughout the earth to **strengthen** those whose hearts are **fully** committed to him."*

2 Corinthians 12:10: *"Since I know it is all for Christ's good, I am quite content with my weaknesses and with insults, hardships, persecutions, and calamities. For when I am **weak**, then I am **strong**."*

CHAPTER 3

John 3:16: *"For God so **loved** the world that he gave his only Son, so that everyone who **believes** in him will not perish but have eternal life."*

Hebrews 13:5b: *"… because God has said, 'Never will I **leave** you; never will I **forsake** you.'"*

CHAPTER 4

1 Thessalonians 5:16-19 (NLT): *"Always be joyful. Always keep on **praying**. No matter what happens, always be thankful, for this is God's **will** for you who belong to Christ Jesus. Do not defile the Holy Spirit."*

Psalm 139:17-18 (NLT): *"How precious it is, Lord, to realize that you are thinking about me **constantly**! I can't even count how many times a day your thoughts turn towards me. And when I awaken in the morning, you are still thinking of **me**!"*

Deuteronomy 17:19-20 (NLT): *"That copy of the laws shall be his constant companion. He must read from it every day of his life so that he will learn to respect the Lord his God by **obeying** all of his commands. This regular **reading** of God's laws will prevent him from feeling that he is better than is fellow citizens. It will also prevent him from turning away from God's laws in the slightest respect, and will ensure his having a long, good reign. His sons will then follow him upon the throne."*

CHAPTER 5

2 Thessalonians 1:9 (NLT): *"They will be punished in everlasting hell, forever **separated** from the Lord, never to see the glory of his power."*

Revelation 12:9 (NLT): *"This great dragon – the ancient serpent called the devil, or **Satan**, the one deceiving the whole world – was thrown down onto the earth with all his **army**."*

James 4:7 (NLT): *"So give yourselves humbly to God. Resist the devil and he will **flee** from you."*

CHAPTER 6

James 1:2-4 (NLT): *"Dear brothers, is your life full of difficulties and temptations? Then be happy, for when the way is rough, your patience has a chance to **grow**. So let it grow, and don't try to squirm out of your problems. For when your patience is finally in full bloom, then you will be ready for anything, strong in character, full and **complete**."*

1 Peter 3:17 (TRSV): *"For it's better to suffer for doing right, if that should be God's **will**, then for doing wrong."*

Mark 8:34-35 (NLT): "*Then he called his disciples and the crowds to come over and listen. 'If any of you wants to be my follower,' he told them, 'you must put aside your own pleasures and shoulder your cross, and follow me closely. If you insist on saving your life, you will **lose** it. Only those who throw away their lives for my sake and for the sake of the Good News will ever know what it means to really **live**."*

CHAPTER 7

1 Corinthians 11:3: *"Now I want you to realize that the head of every man is Christ, and the head of the woman is **man**, and the head of Christ is **God**."*

CHAPTER 8

Psalm 34:18-10 (NLT): *"The Lord is close to those whose hearts are breaking; he rescues those who are **humbly** sorry for their sins. The good man does not escape all troubles – he has them too. But the Lord helps him in each and every one."*

Ephesians 4:31-32: *"Get rid of all **bitterness**, rage and anger, brawling and slander, along with every form of malice. Be kind and compassionate to one another, forgiving each other, just as in Christ God forgave you."*

Colossians 3:13: *"Bear with each other and **forgive** whatever grievances you may have against one another. Forgive as the Lord **forgave** you."*

CHAPTER 9

Hebrews 10:36: *"You need to persevere so that when you have done the **will** of God, you will receive what he has promised."*

Galatians 6:2: *"Carry each other's **burdens**, and in this way you will fulfill the law of Christ."*

CHAPTER 10

1 Corinthians 12:4-11: *"There are different kinds of **gifts**, but the same Spirit. There are different kinds of service, but the same Lord. There are different kinds of working, but the same God works all of them in all men. Now to each one the manifestation of the Spirit is given for the common good. To one there is given through the Spirit the message of wisdom, to another the message of knowledge by means of the same Spirit, to another faith by the same Spirit, to another gifts of healing by that one Spirit, to another miraculous powers, to another prophecy, to another distinguishing between spirits, to another speaking in different kinds of tongues, and to still another the interpretation of tongues. All these are the work of one and the same Spirit, and he gives them to each one, just as he **determines**."*

Matthew 6:34: *"Therefore do not worry about **tomorrow**, for tomorrow will worry about itself. Each day has enough trouble of its own."*

CHAPTER 11

Psalm 18:35: *"You gave me your **shield** of victory, and your right **hand** sustains me; you stoop down to make me great.*

Matthew 6:33 (NLT): *"So don't be anxious about tomorrow. God will take care of your tomorrow too. Live one **day** at a time."*

8/06